Nurse Prescribing

Nurse Prescribing

Edited by Jennifer L. Humphries and Joyce Green

MACMILLAN

First published 1999 by
MACMILLAN PRESS LTD
Houndmills, Basingstoke, Hampshire RG21 6XS
and London
Companies and representatives throughout the world

ISBN 0-333-72611-1

A catalogue record for this book is available from the British Library.

This book is printed on paper suitable for recycling and made from fully managed and sustained forest sources.

10 9 8 7 6 5 4 3 2
08 07 06 05 04 03 02 01 00 99

Editing and origination by
Aardvark Editorial, Mendham, Suffolk

Printed and bound in Great Britain by
Antony Rowe Ltd, Chippenham, Wiltshire

To Steve, Tristam and Geraint

Contents

Notes on Contributors

Rosalyn Anderson BSc(Hons), DipTherMR, PharmS

Independent Pharmaceutical Advisor, Lorac Clinical Pharmacy Services, Cheadle, Cheshire

Ros undertakes prescribing reviews within primary care for GPs and community and practice nurses. She works jointly with nurse practitioners on anticoagulant and medication review clinics, is involved in training nurse prescribers from the initial pilot work in Bolton and subsequently, and has analysed nurse prescribing data for the Department of Health. She has also lectured to a variety of health professionals on the prescribing of wound care, incontinence and stoma products, and has written bulletins on these topics for the National Prescribing Centre.

Lorraine Berry RGN, DipHV

Health Visitor/Nurse Practitioner, Community Healthcare, Bolton NHS Trust

Lorraine qualified as a health visitor at the same time as the pilot for nurse prescribing commenced in Bolton. As an experienced nurse prescriber, she has addressed many conferences on the subject. She has participated in the nurse prescribing course at Manchester Metropolitan University by sharing her skills and experiences with student nurse prescribers. She works with a GP practice in a dual role as health visitor and nurse practitioner, and is a skilled speaker.

Mark Campbell MPhil, MRPharmS

NHS Executive Northern and Yorkshire Regional Drugs and Therapeutics Centre, Newcastle upon Tyne

Mark Campbell is Prescribing Unit Manager in the Regional Drug and Therapeutics Centre, Newcastle upon Tyne, which undertakes a wide range of work on prescribing and therapeutics on behalf of the Northern and Yorkshire Regional Office of the NHS Executive, including performance management, new drug evaluation, analysis and research.

Joyce Green MA, BA, RN, RM, RHV, QN, NDNCert, RNT, DNT

Part-time Lecturer, Department of Health Care Studies, Manchester Metropolitan University

Joyce has been involved with community nurse education for many years and has been a course leader for both district nursing and practice nursing. She is currently joint course leader for the nurse prescribing course and was a member of the ENB Nurse Prescribing Steering Group. She was involved in the writing of the current course and participated in satelliting the approved course at Manchester Metropolitan University to seven other institutions in the third phase of the introduction of nurse prescribing. She has recently been a member of the ENB Working Group (1997/98) revising the Nurse Prescribing Open Learning Pack.

Eileen Groves MA (Health Care Ethics), RN, DN, DNT, RNT, CertEd

Senior Lecturer, Department of Health Care Studies, Manchester Metropolitan University

Eileen is lecturer in health care ethics and law and also teaches law and politics at the university. She is chair of a local research ethics committee.

Jennifer Humphries MA, BSc(Hons), RN, RM, RHV, RHVT, CertEd

Senior Lecturer, Department of Primary and Community Nursing, University of Central Lancashire

Jennifer has been teaching in community nurse education for the past 8 years. She was involved in developing and delivering the nurse prescribing course and, with Joyce Green, participated in satelliting the approved course at Manchester Metropolitan University to seven other institutions in the third phase of the introduction of nurse prescribing.

Rita Hurst SRN, NDNCert

District Nursing Sister, Community Healthcare, Bolton NHS Trust

Rita has been a district nurse for 17 years. She became one of the first community nurses in the country to prescribe when the GP practice she worked with was chosen as one of the eight pilot sites in 1994. She has addressed many conferences and is an experienced speaker on the subject of nurse prescribing. She has recently been part of the ENB Working Group (1997/98) revising the Nurse Prescribing Open Learning Pack.

Joel Richman BA, MA(Econ), PhD

Joel is a founder member of Manchester Polytechnic, now the Manchester Metropolitan University. Publications include: Traffic Wardens: An Ethnography of Street Administration *(Manchester University Press, 1983),* Medicine and Health *(Longman, 1987) and* Health *(Macmillan, 1992). He has made contributions to several edited books and journals. Before retirement, Joel was awarded a chair in medical sociology and anthropology. As emeritus professor, he continues to work part time in the Department of Health Care Studies at Manchester Metropolitan University.*

David Skidmore MSc, PhD, RN, DipN, CertEd, DipPE

Head of Department of Health Care Studies, Manchester Metropolitan University

David was a community psychiatric nurse and behavioural therapist in the early 1970s prior to taking up full-time study in medical sociology. He subsequently fell into an academic career and has been involved with community nursing research for some 25 years. His interest in the education and development of nursing practice had its genesis in community research in the 1980s, and he has been actively involved in this field of research ever since.

Foreword

In 1986 I started what was to become the long haul to allow nurses to prescribe. It seemed logical, sensible and fairly easy to achieve. A survey of community nurses conducted in 1985 showed that 30 per cent cleaned the surgery and for GPs the most important job of the nurse was to fill his or her bag. Nurse prescribing became a giant cultural hurdle to turn handmaidens into autonomous practitioners.

While there was enthusiam for the project from many nurses and doctors, others found the change difficult, not least the Treasury, many politicians and parts of the NHS establishment. It was part of the feminist revolution which was being fought in every walk of life from the Church of England to cricket clubs. Nurse prescribing triggered a wholesale reassessment of the role of nurses, their training and the move to a profession qualified with degrees in nursing.

The transition has not been easy; long delays, primary legislation and dealing with the implications for nearly half a million nurses. We are now at the stage where all community nurses are or will soon be able to prescribe, and the move towards enabling all specialist nurses to take that responsibility is unstoppable.

It is a quiet, continuing revolution which must not lose its momentum, because it not only strengthens team work but does so much to improve health care to all the people of this country.

BARONESS CUMBERLEGE

Preface

Nurse prescribing is an innovative project which has government support and, although at the time of writing it is restricted to those district nurses and health visitors who have undergone specialised training, the aim of this book is to provide access to a range of perspectives on nurse prescribing and to promote discourse on these issues. It takes a critical look at the development and implications of nurse prescribing, discussing features relating to patients and clients, the nurses themselves and the nursing profession in general. Relevant professional issues are examined and comprehensively reviewed within the framework of current community nursing practice.

By adopting a broad approach to nurse prescribing, the intention is to appeal to all health care professionals interested in developments in community and primary health care. Although aimed primarily at post-registration community nurses and as a necessary text for all those undertaking a nurse prescribing course, because nurse prescribing is a momentous evolution in nursing practice, we would consider this book to be essential supplementary reading for both student nurses and other post-registration students. The *Scope of Professional Practice* (UKCC, 1992) outlines the need for practice and education to be sensitive, relevant and responsive to the changing needs of patients and clients. Nurse prescribing is one such initiative and it behoves all nurses and health care professionals to be aware of contemporary issues affecting nursing practice and patient/client care.

All the chapters have been written by different authors and because of this readers may perceive variations in style and presentation of material. It has not been our intention to edit out these differences, as each contributor has their own unique body of knowledge and expertise to add to the nurse prescribing discussion. By offering a range of perspectives, this should enrich the content enabling readers, whether current prescribers or not, to consider prescribing in the context of their professional role and to reflect on the implications from both local and national perspectives.

Chapter 1 sets the scene by presenting a historical overview of the nurse prescribing initiative within a legislative framework, outlining the development of the training programme and indicating how nurse prescribing fits in with contemporary community nursing practice.

Chapter 2 covers the very important issues of ethical and legal principles and accountability.

In Chapter 3 assessment and evaluation strategies are discussed in some detail and the arguments presented clearly demonstrate how these strategies can be applied to nurse prescribing and assist community nurses in the decision-making process.

Chapter 4 offers a rich source of practical information on the responsibilities of prescribing including guidance for prescription writing, generic prescribing and independent reference sources for prescribers.

Chapter 5 discusses some of the financial implications of prescribing and the ways in which nurse prescribing is being monitored. Some national and international perspectives are also considered.

Chapter 6 focuses on non-compliance and who is the non-compliant patient. A review of the extensive research in this area, although naturally medically based, has much to offer prescribing nurses and is intended to increase awareness and stimulate debate.

The reality of nurse prescribing is illustrated in Chapter 7 through the experiences of prescribing nurses participating in the demonstration project. Case examples of prescribing situations are included, focusing the reader on some of the pertinent issues that nurse prescribing raises and enabling reflection on current practice.

Chapter 8 takes a considered look at the extended role of the nurse by analysing the role of specialist practitioners and putting nurse prescribing as the central focus of this debate. This poses many questions about which nurses should be able to prescribe, how far the nurse's role should progress, the benefits for patients/clients and the implications for the nursing profession. The intention is to provoke the reader to take a critical look at nursing and the possible implications of extending the scope of clinical practice.

The final chapter, Chapter 9, examines the most recent developments that have occurred in the sphere of nurse prescribing. It also looks at current issues and considers some possible future implications for nursing practice.

The nurse prescribing initiative is a changing one and the Crown Reviews report (DoH, 1998) has addressed the issue of group protocols. At the time of writing we are eagerly awaiting the next report of the working group chaired by June Crown set up by the government to review prescribing, supply and administration of medicines. It is hoped that this group, who are considering the future of nurse prescribing alongside other prescribing issues, will indicate the way forward for nurses and the further development of the nurse prescribing project.

The text set out to be an edited compilation of practical and theoretical perspectives relating to nurse prescribing, supported by reference to relevant reading and research. We hope that we have achieved our objective and that readers will find it both interesting and informative.

REFERENCES

Department of Health (1998) *Review of Prescribing, Supply and Administration of Medicines: A Report on the Supply and Administration Under Group Protocols*. DoH, London.
UKCC (1992) *Scope of Professional Practice*. UKCC, London.

1 Development of the nurse prescribing initiative

Joyce Green

Nurse prescribing is a comparatively new and exciting development for the nursing profession, the vision of community nurses and health visitors being able to prescribe for patients having begun in 1986. This chapter will incorporate a historical overview of the nurse prescribing initiative and include reference to relevant reports and legislation, a brief summary of the pilot sites and how the current training for nurse prescribing developed. Issues relating to teamwork in primary health care, including community profiling and case load management, and the circumstances in which a nurse may prescribe, will be addressed in order to illustrate how nurse prescribing fits in with the current role of community nursing and health visiting.

A historical overview of the legislative framework

According to Blatt (1997), nurse prescribing is not a new idea but was first recommended by the Royal College of Nursing (RCN) in 1980, and became part of the government's policy agenda in 1986 with the Cumberlege Report. A team, chaired by Julia Cumberlege, was appointed in June 1985, its terms of reference being as follows:

> To study the nursing services provided outside hospital by Health Authorities, and to report to the Secretary of State on how resources can be used more effectively, so as to improve the services available to client groups. The input from nurses employed by general practitioners will be taken into account.
>
> (DHSS 1986)

The Review Team were asked to report to the Secretary of State by the end of the year so had 6 months in which to gather and collate their evidence. During this period, district nurses indicated that, based on a full nursing assessment of the patients' individual health care needs, they were constantly recommending to general practitioners (GPs) the need for particular dressings or appliances for patients. However, they had to get the GPs to sanction and sign the prescription, which was felt to be very time-wasting. In addition, according to Cumberlege (DHSS 1986), many nurses had also become very skilled in managing pain relief for terminally ill patients.

The following recommendation was included in the Report:

> that the DHSS should agree a limited list of items and simple agents which may be prescribed by nurses as part of a nursing care programme, and issue guidelines to enable nurses to control drug dosage in well-defined circumstances.
>
> (DHSS 1986)

This recommendation and its implications were subsequently reviewed by the Department of Health (DoH) advisory group chaired by Dr June Crown.

The Crown Report, published in 1989 (DoH 1989), recommended that suitably qualified nurses working in the community, defined as those nurses with a district nurse or health visitor qualification, should be authorised to prescribe in defined circumstances from a limited list of items to be included in the *Nurse Prescribers' Formulary* (NPF) (see Appendix 1). They also recommended that nurses should be able to supply medicines within group protocols or adjust their timing and dosage within patient-specific protocols. These protocol issues were not taken further, and, according to Jones and Gough (1997), 'in the light of the current widespread use of protocols and their questionable legality, this can be viewed only as a lost opportunity'.

Subsequently, Mr Roger Simms, Member of Parliament for Chislehurst, introduced a Private Members Bill making legislative provision for nurse prescribing; this received Royal Assent in March 1992. Since then, much preparatory work has been undertaken in order to ensure that nurse prescribing can be implemented in an efficient and cost-effective way. The primary legislation that permits initial nurse prescribing is the Medicinal Products: Prescription by Nurses Act 1992, but, although this Act was passed in 1992, the necessary secondary legislation, Medicinal Prescription by Nurses etc. (Commencement No. 1) Order 1994, did not come into effect until 3 October 1994.

Developing the initiative: the demonstration sites

On 21 November 1993, Baroness Cumberlege announced the introduction of demonstration sites for nurse prescribing, the purpose of the demonstration sites being to explore how the clinical, managerial and financial aspects of nurse prescribing could be managed effectively. GP fundholders and community units who could demonstrate commitment to nurse prescribing submitted a proforma to the DoH giving information about their unit and the fundholding practice. This was jointly signed by the practice, the community provider, the Family Health Service Authority and the region.

The selection criteria for the demonstration sites included:

- evidence of an established GP fundholding practice
- a well-established primary health care team
- a contract for community services with a provider unit
- practice computing systems to enable a linkage of patient and prescribing data
- the adequacy of management information systems
- a willingness to participate in data collection/evaluation prior to, during and after implementation
- the provision of representation on an implementation group and modification of the existing contract if necessary.

Eight sites were chosen, one in each of the health regions in England. The sites included inner city, rural and urban practices, some with large elderly populations and some with large numbers of children, especially under 5s. Implementation in the eight demonstration sites was achieved by April 1994. The whole project was subject to an independent, fully researched evaluation, which began in May 1994, to enable 'before and after' comparisons to be made. The University of Liverpool was commissioned to provide a qualitative evaluation of patient, nurse and doctor satisfaction with the scheme, and an analysis of the cost–benefit aspects of the scheme was undertaken by the University of York.

Two colleges of higher education (one in the north and one in the south of England) were invited to provide the taught component of the nurse prescribing course, and each submitted a detailed course document for validation by the English National Board for Nursing, Midwifery and Health Visiting (ENB) in August 1994. After completing the ENB Open Learning Pack on nurse prescribing (ENB 1994), nurses and health visitors in the prescribing sites attended one of these ENB-approved courses during September 1994 in readiness for commencing their nurse prescribing role in October 1994.

According to Jones and Gough (1997), 'with only eight sites involved, data from the project were not of sufficient statistical significance to extrapolate to the outcome of a national expansion of nurse prescribing'. Therefore in 1996, Bolton, one of the original pilot sites, was expanded to include 60 more practices, and a further 150 community nurses were trained as nurse prescribers. Two pilot sites were designated in Scotland in the same year. In 1997, following the publication of the White Paper *Primary Care: Delivering the Future* (DoH 1996), a further seven pilot sites in NHS Trusts were inaugurated in England, and the Bolton site has also been further extended to include Wigan. A press release in July 1997 announced that 'plans to extend nurse prescribing to Wales were unveiled as part of a package of primary health care measures announced by Welsh health minister Win Griffiths' (Scott 1997). This announcement appears to have received a very positive response from Welsh nurses, who were disappointed at being left out of the original pilot scheme.

Preparation for nurse prescribing: education and training

In July 1991, the United Kingdom Central Council for Nursing, Midwifery and Health Visiting (UKCC) responded to the DoH's invitation to establish the standard, kind and content of educational preparation for nurse prescribing. It was recognised that the training should enable district nurses and health visitors to meet the learning outcomes set by the UKCC in order for them to prescribe safely and effectively from an appropriate knowledge base. According to the UKCC (1991), 'in order to complete the preparation for nurse prescribing, individuals will need to ensure that they have sufficient knowledge of relevant pharmacology and therapeutics to enable them to undertake the programme. The Nurses' Formulary would provide the basis for identification of requirements.' The previous education and training of the course participants would also influence the type and length of programme required, in particular the amount of pre-course preparation necessary. The kind of programme envisaged by the UKCC would fall into two categories:

> a free standing module for district nurses and health visitors who are already qualified – and preparation which could be incorporated into the curriculum for district nursing and health visiting from a date agreed by the council.
>
> (UKCC 1991)

A newsletter for institutions of higher education, issued by the ENB in July 1992, outlined the progress made with regard to the educational requirements for nurse prescribing. The following statement was incorporated:

> to ensure the availability of a suitable programme leading to the achievement of competence and authority to prescribe, the ENB has been given responsibility and funding for developing and delivering:
>
> ● an open learning pack
> ● a video
> ● guidance for the validation of programmes to be presented by institutions of higher education currently offering district nurse and health visitor courses.
>
> (ENB 1992)

A Steering Group with DoH and higher education representation was set up in order to monitor and guide the preparation and development of the above. In order to ensure that the most effective strategies were employed, the Steering Group held a number of regional consultation days with district nurse and health visitor course leaders, formed a Working Group to plan and supervise the production of the open learning pack and appointed open learning consultants to advise the group and develop the materials. As stated in the ENB newsletter (1992), the Working Group represented 'the major stakeholders in the process of preparing district nurses and health visitors for prescribing: practitioners, managers, lecturers, ENB directorate and the Department of Health'. The Group provided a wide range of professional expertise and also knowledge and experience of open learning.

The learning outcomes defined by the UKCC are:

- the ability to prescribe safely, effectively and cost-effectively from the Nurses' Formulary;
- an understanding of the potential side effects of, and reactions to, the items in the Nurses' Formulary;
- an understanding of the team and individual roles of doctors, dentists and pharmacists in relation to prescribing;
- an understanding of the requirements of the legislation relevant to the practice of nurse prescribing and
- an understanding of accountability and professional responsibility in relation to nurse prescribing.

> UKCC response to the Department of Health standard, kind and content of educational preparation for Nurse Prescribing
> (UKCC 30 July 1991, Section 5, p. 2)

One of the Working Group's main tasks was, based on the UKCC learning outcomes, to devise more specific outcomes for the open learning pack. These were considered further in the light of information received from colleagues on the consultation days and from practitioner profiles taken from telephone interviews. It was decided that, in order to ensure integration of the open learning pack and the taught component of the course, most topic areas should be included in both, the open learning pack forming the bridge leading from the individual's current experience into the taught component. This would enable course participants to apply their existing knowledge and practice to nurse prescribing issues and to identify their own individual learning needs, which could be addressed in the taught part of the course.

The open learning pack is divided into the following areas of study: getting to grips with nurse prescribing, accountability, prescribing safely and effectively, ethical issues, prescribing in a team context, administrative arrangements and evaluating effectiveness. These topics are further developed using a variety of teaching methods, including the ENB video, during the taught course and these trigger much discussion and debate. In addition, the taught course also includes relevant pharmacology and therapeutics based on the NPF, together with other legal, financial and practical aspects of nurse prescribing.

The necessary training for nurse prescribing was outlined in the UKCC's response to an invitation from the DoH in July 1991. At that time, a 2-day taught course component was recommended, but, following evaluations from the initial courses held in September 1994, the format of this part of the course was modified. As stated in paragraph 3.2 of the NHS Executive's *Nurse Prescribing Guidance* (1997), the current model of training consists of two parts. The first part consists of the ENB Open Learning Pack (ENB 1994), which students work through in their own time prior to attending the taught course, although local arrangements for study time may be made with the approval of the nurse's employer. This package will take 10–20 hours to work through depending on the nurse's prior knowledge and experience. The 3-day taught component is taken at a college of higher education that already provides district nurse and health visitor education and is followed up by a half-day return to sit the examination. At present, nurses can only qualify by attending an ENB-approved course.

The UKCC (1991) stated that 'a variety of assessment strategies should be employed to test knowledge and synthesis and the application of theory to practice. Assessment should focus upon the principles of nurse prescribing, and the professional accountability and responsibility of the nurse undertaking the role.' Several assessment strategies were considered, including written examination, self-assessment, case study analysis, peer assessment, keeping a reflective journal and a defined period of supervised practice. However, as a matter of expediency, partly due to the tight timescale and the need to identify quickly whether course members were competent to prescribe in practice, the written examination was chosen. Most educationalists, given the essentially practical nature of nurse prescribing, would have preferred a combination of the other options, but the written examination, which is divided into two parts, has proved to be a satisfactory method of assessment, for the following reasons. First, the short answer questions, some of which are multiple choice, are a useful way of ensuring a wide coverage of the curriculum and testing the principles of nurse prescribing. Second, the context-dependent questions based on case study analysis test knowledge of the nurse's role in prescribing situations and the understanding and application of identifying an appropriate rationale for decision-making in respect of nurse prescribing.

Assessment strategies may change in the future as the nurse prescribing initiative is developed further and eventually becomes an integral part of district nurse and health visitor education. Also, if current legislation is changed to include other branches of nursing, course content, length of training and assessment may need to be reviewed in order to ensure that all nurses are prepared for their nurse prescribing role in the most appropriate manner. Now that there is a nucleus of experienced nurse prescribers across the country, it will probably be easier to adopt a method of assessment that more accurately reflects practice, as there are nurses and health visitors who could act as mentors/supervisors for those undertaking training. Indeed, nurse prescribing training is subject to ongoing evaluation and review, and, as stated in paragraph 3.3 of the NHS Executive's *Nurse Prescribing Guidance* (1997), 'In an effort to reduce infrastructure costs while maintaining the quality of training, further training models will be developed during the pilot trials and evaluated.' The ongoing monitoring and evaluation of the examination procedure has enabled the strengths and weaknesses of the system to be identified and minor modifications to be made. This knowledge will also help to ensure that an informed choice is made if and when the assessment strategy is changed or modified in the future.

Nurse prescribing and primary health care

Primary health care services are the first point of contact for most patients and their families, and are the most frequently used within the National Health Service. The skills, expertise, and knowledge base of all those who work in primary care have developed to meet challenges created by an increasingly more informed public, advances in technology, and better service outcomes.

(Poulton 1997, p. 1)

The role of nurses and health visitors in primary health care has developed to meet the changing health care needs of the population, and community nurses currently have a vital role to play in a primary care-led NHS. Nurse prescribing has an important contribution to make in improving the service to patients and clients within the primary health care context. In fact, the potential advantages and benefits of nurse prescribing were clearly identified in the Crown Report (DoH 1989) and included an improvement in patient care as nurses would be able to manage a patient's condition more effectively, a better use of patients' and nurses' time, thus enabling patients to receive treatment with the minimum of delay, and a clarification of professional responsibilities, which would strengthen professional partnership within the primary health care team.

The nurse or health visitor responsible for the programme of care for the patient or client is uniquely placed to make an accurate assessment of his or her needs based on a critical professional appraisal. For those nurses and health visitors who are trained as nurse prescribers, prescribing issues are an integral part of that assessment, and they utilise their clinical and professional judgement to decide when it is necessary to prescribe and which products from the NPF are the most appropriate to meet the needs identified. Community profiling and workload analysis will also enable nurses and health visitors to identify those patient/client groups and individuals most likely to require nurse-initiated prescriptions. Nurse prescribing will also impinge on the nurse's teaching and health promotion role. For example, patients experiencing problems with constipation may require advice about diet, fluid intake and variations in bowel habits, which will still be a first-line strategy in most cases; now, however, following a full clinical assessment, the nurse will be able to prescribe an appropriate laxative if this is necessary. The nurse is also in an ideal position to advise the patient on the action of the medication prescribed and to plan appropriate follow-up and evaluation of the situation for the care plan.

Have the potential benefits been realised in practice? It would appear so as, according to Luker *et al.* (1997a), 'the advantages patients identified coincided with the anticipated benefits, while the disadvantages that had been anticipated before the study were not confirmed' (p. 51). From the results of the study undertaken, it would appear that patients did receive treatment more promptly, and this was of great benefit to themselves and their carers. Luker *et al.* (1997a) also state that 'although it was

anticipated that district nurses' patients would be the main bene-
ficiaries of nurse prescribing, health visitor clients, in particular,
were more likely to mention the increased convenience; practice
nurses' patients, while benefiting overall, noted fewer changes'
(p. 54). These opinions reflected the relative ease or difficulty
that each of these groups of patients had in obtaining a prescription before nurse prescribing. The reaction from patients and
clients was extremely positive, and in some instances the nurse
was cited as being the preferred prescriber. Patients quickly
familiarised themselves with the nurses' remit, and there did not
appear to be any undue confusion surrounding the nurses' and
doctors' role in prescribing. According to Luker *et al.* (1997a),
'patients were conscious of the fact that in the past the nurse had
made the decision but the prescription had to be obtained from
the GP. For these nurses this anomaly has now been rectified'
(p. 54). The NHS Executive HQ *Nurse Prescribing Guidance*
April 1997 very clearly states in section 7 the circumstances in
which nurses may prescribe; these are cited in Appendix 2 of
this book.

Most nurses and health visitors participating in the demonstration sites also had a positive reaction to nurse prescribing. The
main benefits appear to be increased job satisfaction, time-saving
and improved patient or client care, while the main frustration is
the limited nature of the nurse's formulary, some nurses wanting
to see additional items added to the list. It is also possible that, as
the nurses are more aware of costs, this may result in some cost
savings. According to the Executive Summary of the *Evaluation of
Nurse Prescribing Final Report* (Luker *et al.* 1997b):

> there has been little reported change in professional relationships,
> between primary health care team members, with the notable exception
> of the pharmacist. District nurses reported a closer relationship with the
> pharmacist, HVs and PNs, who previously had very little, if any, contact
> now do have contact; this they have reported as being a positive aspect
> of nurse prescribing.
>
> (pp. 12–13)

Also cited in this document is the fact that many professionals
included in the evaluation indicated many advantages of nurse
prescribing for patients and for the primary health care team.
Time-saving was frequently mentioned; over half the GPs had

noticed that nurse prescribing was saving them time and that they were signing fewer nurse-generated prescriptions, but in most cases this was not quantifiable. According to the ENB Open Learning Pack (1994), teamwork is an essential part of nurse prescribing, and even those nurses working independently will have to report back to their nurse manager and have the opportunity to discuss their workload with other nurses and health visitors. For some practice nurses, this may not be quite so easy, and therefore the importance of the advantages of an integrated primary health care team, whose members have common goals and understand and respect each other's role and function within the team, cannot be overemphasised. Communication and teamwork are essential for effective nurse prescribing, one way of ensuring clear communication being to use well-defined local policies and/or protocols. In the interests of good patient or client care, it also important to maintain good relationships with those nurses in the team who are unable to prescribe and keep them informed about any developments of the nurse prescribing initiative.

Nurse prescribing – a changing role?

The final report of the Crown Review Committee's deliberation relating to nurse prescribing is, as yet, unknown, although one can speculate on possible outcomes and developments. According to Bradley (1997):

> the government intention, declared in recent white papers on primary care, is to roll out the nurse prescribing scheme to cover the whole country. All this would appear to imply that nurse prescribing has now arrived and is about to transform life for nurses, GPs and their patients. Well, don't you believe it. Unless the constraints currently operating on nurse prescribing are radically altered, the ability of nurses to prescribe will only ever have a very limited impact. The reasons for this are that nurse prescribing is confined to a restricted group of nurses (with district nursing or health visitor qualifications who have undergone further specific training) and to a fairly narrow formulary of drugs and appliances, most of which are available without prescription anyway. The result of these restrictions are that the majority of nurses who would like the power to prescribe that is, practice nurses without the necessary qualifications, cannot do so. Furthermore, many of the items nurses

would like to be able to prescribe, particularly those that enhance their role in chronic disease management, for example in asthma and diabetes, are precluded.

However, although there are advocates for extending the NPF, there are also those who have expressed concern about nurses' knowledge of items already included in the formulary. Some of these points are also borne out by Luker *et al.* (1997c), who state that, since the publication of the Crown Report (DoH 1989), considerable changes have taken place in the role of nurses working in the community. This particularly applies to practice nurses, whose role is very diverse and has developed considerably since the implementation of the GP contract (DoH 1989b). Atkin *et al.* (1993), in a national consensus of practice nurses, identified that about 96 per cent of practice nurses were involved in the provision of immunisations, almost 30 per cent in family planning, 55 per cent in diabetes management and 52 per cent in asthma management. The extension of the practice nurse's role has led to much discussion on whether the nurses' formulary is too restrictive, especially in relation to chronic disease management, for example care of the asthmatic patient.

Practice nurses who have undergone further specific training and obtained the Diploma in Asthma Care may be running nurse-led clinics within the general practice setting and advising patients on the most appropriate medication to control and improve their medical condition, but the nurses are unable to prescribe this medication and currently have to generate a prescription from the GP. This is seen by some nurses to be very frustrating and poten-tially time-wasting. Luker *et al.* (1997c) argue that practice nurses already influence the prescribing behaviour of GPs in the areas of asthma and diabetes, and that the nurses' ability and practice has 'out-stripped' the parameters of the NPF. It is also important to recognise that, if nurses are to take on additional responsibilities in respect of nurse prescribing, they must be adequately trained and prepared. Luker *et al.* (1997c) point out that, although the role of the practice nurse has expanded, there is a diversity of expertise among this group and considerable variation in the qualifications they possess. According to Atkin *et al.* (1993), fewer than half the practice nurses had attended a practice nurse course validated by a national board for nursing, midwifery and health visiting, and only

12 per cent held a district nurse certificate and 3.3 per cent a health visitor qualification, which is currently a prerequisite to be a nurse prescriber. Atkin *et al.* (1993) also noted that a number of nurses also expressed a need for training in areas related to practice nurse practice, including immunisations (11 per cent), asthma (38 per cent), family planning (39 per cent) and diabetes (42 per cent). This reinforces the point that it is essential for all nurses to be properly and appropriately trained before undertaking additional professional responsibilities. If the remit of nurse prescribing is extended in the future, variations in preparation for practice, of which practice nursing is an example, will need to be considered when planning the future education of nurse prescribers.

Despite the positive evaluation of the nurse prescribing initiative, Luker *et al.* (1997c) state that:

> there was concern about the limited nature of the NPF, for health visitors and practice nurses in particular, as it did not have direct applicability to their areas of work. This was reflected in the relative infrequency with which these nurses prescribed when compared with district nurses. Consequently many of the benefits anticipated for nurses had not materialised for them, and they still depended on GPs to authorise prescriptions.

The Crown Report (DoH 1989) did, however, envisage that there would be developments in the role of nurses and advocated regular reviews of the contents of the NPF. At the time of writing, a Working Group chaired by June Crown, set up by the government to review the prescribing, supply and administration of medicines, is expected to complete its task in December 1998. Nurse prescribing is included in their deliberations, and it is hoped that many of the issues highlighted by the *Evaluation of Nurse Prescribing Final Report* (Luker *et al.* 1997b), and any concerns and evidence submitted by various professional bodies and individuals, will be considered and addressed. The outcome of these discussions and any subsequent recommendations is awaited with interest.

Conclusion

In spite of its critics, nurse prescribing is a major step forward for nurses, one which has, in the main, been met with a very positive and enthusiastic response, having been seen to have strengthened teamwork in primary care in some instances. Patients appear to have welcomed the initiative, and GPs and pharmacists have been very supportive. The Crown Report (1989) indicated a number of benefits that could arise out of nurse prescribing, including an improvement in patient care; a better use of the patients' and nurses' time, and the clarification of professional responsibilities, leading to improved communication between team members. The report also stressed the uniqueness of the community nurses' role in that they are well versed in the needs of each patient or client and in the services and resources available to help meet those needs. This knowledge and experience enables them to provide a service tailored to individual needs and circumstances. Nurse prescribing is now, for some nurses, an integral and important part of this clinical care.

Let us hope that the current demonstration sites are only the beginning, but, as Jones and Gough (1997) state:

> for nurse prescribing to find full expression appropriate to the demands of today's health services and the expanding nature of nursing practice, the existing legislation needs urgent revision.
>
> (p. 42)

They advocate the lifting of restrictions on the type of nurse able to prescribe and the expansion of the nurses' formulary. In the light of the ongoing current review looking at the prescribing practices of all health professionals, the RCN, according to Jones and Gough (1997), is:

> working to ensure that the final recommendations of the review acknowledge the coming of age of nursing and nurses' ability to provide highly expert, flexible and appropriate services to their patients in a variety of clinical settings.
>
> (p. 42)

Nurses and health visitors currently able to prescribe acknowledge that nurse prescribing is very much an integral part of their role, and hope that this aspect of their work will continue as it is enabling them to provide a more comprehensive service and gives them increased job satisfaction. Their aim is to treat all patients and clients in an holistic way based on relevant, up-to-date clinical research, and, with the increased emphasis on primary care in the NHS, nurse prescribing is perceived by many to be a valued component of community nursing that will hopefully continue to be part of any new and exciting developments.

References

Atkin, K., Lunt, N., Park, G. and Hirst, M. (1993) *Nurse Count: A National Census of Practice Nurses.* Social Policy Research Unit, York.

Blatt, B. (1997) Nurse prescribing: are you ready? *Practice Nursing* **8**(12): 11–13.

Bradley, C. (1997) Nurse prescribing – unlikely to transform our lives. *Prescriber*, 5 May: 13.

DHSS (1986) *Neighbourhood Nursing – a Focus for Care* (Cumberlege Report). HMSO, London.

DoH (1989) *Report of The Advisory Group on Nurse Prescribing* (Crown Report). HMSO, London.

DoH (1996) *Primary Care: Delivering the Future.* HMSO, London.

ENB (1992) *Nurse Prescribing: Newsletter for Institutions of Higher Education.* ENB, London.

ENB (1994) *Nurse Prescribing. Open Learning Pack.* ENB, London.

Jones, M. and Gough, P. (1997) Nurse prescribing – why has it taken so long? *Nursing Standard* **11**(20): 39–42.

Luker, K.A., Austin, L., Hogg, C., Ferguson, B. and Smith, K. (1997a) Patients' view of nurse prescribing. *Nursing Times* **93**(17): 51–4.

Luker, K.A., Austin, L., Hogg, C. *et al.* (1997b) Evaluation of Nurse Prescribing Final Report: Executive Summary. Unpublished report.

Luker, K.A., Austin, L., Willock, J., Ferguson, B. and Smith, K. (1997c) Nurses' and GPs' views of the nurse prescribers' formulary. *Nursing Standard* **11**(22): 33–8.

NHS Executive HQ (1997) *Nurse Prescribing Guidance, April.* NHSE, Leeds.

Poulton, B. (1997) *Practice Nursing: A Changing Role To Meet Changing Needs.* DoH, London.

Scott, G. (1997) Welsh nurses elated as prescribing arrives. *Nursing Standard* **11**(44): 9.

UKCC (1991) *The Council's Response to the Department of Health's Invitation To Establish the Standard Kind and Content of Educational Preparation for Nurse Prescribing.* UKCC, London.

2

Nurse prescribing – accountability

Eileen Groves

> In my estimation obedience is the first law and very cornerstone of good nursing. And here is the stumbling block for the beginner. No matter how gifted she may be, she will never become a reliable nurse unless she can obey without question. The first and most helpful criticism I received from a doctor was when he told me that I was supposed to be simply an intelligent machine for the purposes of carrying out his orders.
>
> (Dock 1917)

It comes as no surprise to note the date of this much-published quote: such sentiments today would spark widespread reaction and would do little to foster interprofessional relationships between the medical and nursing professions. Yet it has to be remembered that such comment simply reflected the social and gender traditions and ideologies of the era. The nurse in this context was seen as a 'handmaiden' and, as Brown *et al.* (1992) suggest, 'diligent, hardworking, trustworthy and loyal, conscientious in her duties and using her special nurturing skills to provide comfort to patients so that the real work of medicine might not be impeded' (p. 75). Within such an environment, nurses were accountable to the person making decisions regarding patient care, be it the medical practitioner or the management organisation.

Nursing has clearly advanced considerably since then, establishing itself as a profession in its own right with the introduction of the nursing process and nursing models in the 1980s, giving nursing its own unique body of knowledge, and documents from the UKCC, for example the *Code of Professional Conduct* (1992a) and the *Scope of Professional Practice* (1992b), stressing the individual accountability of the nurse. As we are frequently reminded, 'acting on doctor's orders' is no defence in law. Nurses are now expected to act as advocates for patients and clients, and as such may sometimes act in deference to medical colleagues or management.

(Koehn 1994) suggests that the use of the title 'professional' normally applies to those whose work is:

- licensed by the state
- controlled by an organisation which sets standards and ideals
- such that its members have knowledge and skills not normally possessed or understood by the general public
- such that they have autonomy over their work
- of a nature that requires them to have responsibilities and duties to those who need assistance, responsibilities which are not incumbent on others.

It might be argued, then, that it is only in recent years, with the concept of individual accountability, that nurses have truly had the level of autonomy to take on board the title 'professional'.

The advent of nurse prescribing further enhances this notion of autonomy and professional status. The UKCC regulates nursing practice in this country by using the *Code of Professional Conduct* (1992a), as a standard against which criteria for good nursing practice may be set and any allegations of misconduct measured. As a body, the UKCC is statutorily obliged to regulate the standard and practice of its members:

A professional code represents a statement of the role morality of the members of the profession, and in this way professional standards are distinguished from standards imposed by external bodies such as government (although their norms sometimes overlap and agree)

(Beauchamp and Childress 1994, p. 7).

The response to changing health care needs and changing health care provision has greatly increased the scope of practice for the nurse and helped further to develop the professionalisation of nursing and all that such status brings with it, not least individual accountability. Nurse prescribing is one such example of the increase in the scope of practice afforded to suitably qualified nurses, which at the moment includes qualified district nurses, health visitors and practice nurses with a district nurse or health visitor qualification. As nursing practice continues to change, so details of professional accountability may change over time. Accountability is a dynamic process to which nurses will have to adapt and link their individual roles and functions to a set code of professional practice, which will also change over time.

It is not the intention of the author to examine every possible accountability issue that may arise for the nurse prescriber, as individual practice will bring its own range of issues. Neither will it be possible to give definitive answers to the many questions that may be raised – in fact, it is probable that there will be more questions raised than answers offered. It is simply the intention to raise awareness of the extent of accountability in nurse prescribing.

Accountability within the health care professions has assumed a high profile within the past decade as the growth in litigation within health care generally has seen a dramatic rise, health care professionals being held accountable for careless actions or omissions. The notion of accountability is implicit within all elements of the UKCC *Code of Professional Conduct* (1992a) and arises directly out of responsibility. To be accountable, there has to be some authority to act and a basis of knowledge and competency that can be explained and defended:

> Codes of conduct only make sense in the light of accountability. They are only worth something if they can be tested, that is if professionals can be held accountable for decisions and their behaviour.
>
> (ENB 1994)

Tadd (1994) suggests that the concept of professional accountability disregards the fact that not all practitioners are fully autonomous or hold sufficient power in all aspects of their work to be held to account. However, in the area of nurse prescribing, all nurses eligible to prescribe will have power and authority to make prescribing decisions, and as such will be accountable both legally and professionally (ENB 1994).

Nurses who prescribe will be accountable for all aspects of the prescribing process, from the decision to prescribe, to ensuring that the prescription is applied or administered as directed either by the nurse or by the relatives or carers if they are given the medication to administer. This accountability will also include decisions taken in recommending over-the-counter prescriptions and being responsible for the decision not to prescribe:

> The nurse who takes the initial decision and writes the prescription is responsible in law for ensuring that the prescription is used in accordance with the instructions.
>
> (ENB 1994)

Once dispensed, rules governing the safety, storage and administration of drugs, as set out in the UKCC *Standards for the Administration of Medicines* (1992c) and *Standards for Records and Record Keeping* (1993), will apply. Accountability in nursing is clearly not new, and accountability extends to actions, omissions, spheres of influence, delegation or acquiescence in respect of the public, employers and, of course, oneself:

> Ensure that no action or omission on your part, or within your sphere of responsibility, is detrimental to the interests, condition or safety of patients and clients.
>
> (UKCC 1992a, cl. 2)

The *Scope of Professional Practice* (UKCC 1992b) builds on the *Code of Professional Conduct* (UKCC 1992a) and this concept of individual accountability.

As nursing practice continued to develop in the 1980s, and nurses began to undertake 'extended' duties as a matter of course, it was no longer practicable to continue with the system of collecting certificates of competence for 'extended practice'. The *Scope of Professional Practice* was designed to enable nurses to provide continuity of care and holistic care to patients and clients for whom they are responsible. Nurses are no longer expected to collect a wide range of certificates stating their competence to practice, for example in venepuncture or ear syringing, but are asked to make individual decisions regarding their competence to carry out such procedures and be individually accountable for their practice. While it is clearly in patients' interests to have fewer people involved in their care, and it is also in the interests of the personal and professional development of the individual nurse, it does place full responsibility on the nurses to determine the skills required for particular procedures and to ensure that they are appropriately qualified to carry them out. It is therefore incumbent on the individual nurse to ensure that his or her practice is not only safe, but also up to date and research based:

> Acknowledge any limitations in your knowledge and competence and decline any duties or responsibilities unless able to perform them in a safe and skilled manner.
>
> (UKCC 1992a, cl. 4)

Accountability is an integral part of professional practice. As the scope of professional practice continues to widen, nurses are having to make judgements on a wide range of health care issues. Given the increasing emphasis on individual accountability in nursing, it is perhaps pertinent to explore further this concept of accountability from both an ethical and legal perspective, with examples where possible from nurse prescribing practice.

Ethical perspectives

(Please note that the words 'ethical' and 'moral' will be used interchangeably.)

Throughout their lives, people may at some time or other be held accountable for their actions, either legally, morally or simply in a neutral way, to others (Fletcher *et al.* 1995). For example, if we break the law we will be held accountable to the judicial system for our actions; and if we upset or offend someone by our action or inaction, we may be morally accountable for the harm we have caused. Or it may simply be that, in our ordinary, everyday lives, we are accountable to others in a more neutral way for the choices we make about what we do, how we spend our time or how we use our money. In each situation, Fletcher *et al.* (1995) suggest that it may be possible to give reasons for our actions, which will range from very good to none at all.

In health care, ethics and law go hand in hand as the law simply reflects society's views on acceptable ethical standards of practice from health care professionals. A nurse may therefore be held to account both legally and morally for the actions she carries out.

Ethical issues, along with legal issues, in health care have assumed a high profile in recent years, particularly in emotive topic areas such as abortion, in vitro fertilisation and euthanasia, but it is often in ordinary, everyday work situations that nurses face difficult decisions that may have an ethical dimension.

Ethics is concerned with the rights and wrongs of human behaviour, and in health care ethics is about right and wrong actions, and about the responsibilities, obligations and duties we have to patients and clients to ensure that all our actions are right actions. The ethical principles of autonomy and respect for autonomy, beneficence (to do good), non-maleficence (to do no harm) and justice underpin the UKCC *Code of Professional Conduct* (1992a). Such principles, Beauchamp and Childress (1994) maintain, should be easily understood by all health care workers. They also go on to suggest, however, that codes of professional conduct invariably stress rules of do's and don'ts, particularly 'Above all do no harm', rather than the implications of the principles and rules of veracity, respect for autonomy and justice. Codes are particularly concerned with the duties and obligations of professionals within the nurse–patient/client working and caring relationship rather than with any rights of entitlement that the client may have. In recent years, we have seen various rights afforded to citizens, and in health care we have seen the introduction of the *Patient's Charter* (DoH 1992), which highlights those patients' rights which have to be addressed, alongside the professional responsibilities, obligations and duties of the nurse. Resource implications often make it difficult to reconcile the two. Rights automatically imply that someone has a duty to provide for those rights to be fulfilled. Knowing a patient's rights of entitlement and being unable to fulfil those rights creates stress, tension and ethical dilemmas in terms of the fair and just allocation of resources. Ethical rules and principles are complex topics and demand further exploration and discussion outside the remit of this chapter.

Ethical problems arise when there are at least two possible courses of action that can be taken, each of which might bring about the same, or indeed a different, result. Ethical dilemmas occur when we are faced with a situation that appears irresolvable, or if the solution offers alternatives that we find difficult because they may compromise or conflict with our existing moral values of what we feel is a good or right course of action in a particular set of circumstances. Health care professionals are concerned with ensuring that the action they take is right and can be justified against all other possible options, in other words applying what Thompson *et al.* (1994) call 'reasoned judgement'. This requires:

> Skills in assessment of moral situations, informed deliberation on practical and ethical options, ability to act decisively and competently, and critical evaluation of outcomes in terms of cost and benefit.
>
> (p. x)

Other ethical issues may arise as nurses strive to encompass wider role responsibilities to relatives and colleagues, employers and the public. Conflicts may arise for the nurse prescriber in the attitudes and possible resistance of colleagues and other health care professionals to their prescribing role, the expectations of patients and clients, and the questioning of the resource implications in terms of time and finance. In such situations, nurses need to look at how best the patients' interests may be served:

> Act always in such a manner as to promote and safeguard the interests and well-being of patients and clients.
>
> (UKCC 1992a, cl. 1)

Clearly, if the responsibilities within nurse prescribing are to range from decisions of if and when to prescribe, to ensuring correct administration, there may well be ethical dilemmas along the way. The ENB (1994) Nurse Prescribing Open Learning Pack highlights areas that may pose ethical problems or dilemmas for nurses both from within the nurse–patient/client role and in the wider responsibilities that the nurse prescribing role brings.

For example, is there a need to compromise on your choice of prescribed treatment because of local protocol, cost or limited availability in the choice of generic products? Is there patient pressure to prescribe? Will the patient co-operate with an assessment or visit the GP if recommended? If recommending over-the-counter medication, what are the choices available? What can the patient afford? Can the patient afford to pay for medication rather than be given a prescription, thereby possibly releasing monies for others less able to pay? Are there pressures from drug companies and appliance manufacturers to persuade you to prescribe or use their particular products? For example, free trials of a special dressing may produce good results for the patient, but if that dressing is not in the NPF, or is too expensive to continue with once the free supply is ended, what happens then? There are many occasions on which we may be persuaded to try different brands of goods or products in our daily lives, and we all know how convincing such sales talk can be. It would clearly be impossible to read in depth all the research papers regarding new products, but, if we are to apply the maxim 'Above all do no harm', nurses at least need to be aware of any possible or potential side-effects or contraindications of the products they prescribe.

Given all these possible scenarios, how does the nurse choose the right courses of action? Ethical theory would offer many possible ways of looking at the same problem. It would be impracticable here to enter into a great debate and discussion on the various ethical theories and ethical decision-making frameworks that abound, but it is perhaps worth exploring two possible approaches commonly used within health care ethics to illustrate the way in which ethical dilemmas can be approached from differing perspectives.

First, there is the deontological (duty) approach, which suggests that ethical dilemmas are best resolved by taking a duty-based approach to the problem, that is, looking at the problem in terms of what one's duty is to the patient or client and planning a course of action accordingly irrespective of the consequences. Right actions and results are therefore said to be those where one follows one's duty.

The other approach suggests that the right solution to an ethical dilemma will be found in taking actions that will lead to the maximisation of welfare and the greatest good for all concerned (utilitarianism). This is essentially a goal-based or consequentialist approach as one has to have some goal or end in mind in order to direct one's actions to that which maximises welfare and brings about the greater good. An example from nurse prescribing practice that highlights these two differing approaches might be that of a patient whom you have assessed, recognising that a particular brand of cream will be most effective for the speedy healing of his leg ulcer. However, you know that it is extremely expensive, you have a budget to maintain, and you have two other patients still to assess who might also benefit from this cream. Do you take a deontological approach and carry out your duties and responsibilities to the first patient, or do you prescribe a cheaper cream that may take longer to heal the ulcer but with a view of maximising welfare, that is, treating them all for the same cost as it would have been to treat the first person? Or, perhaps worse still, you may be placed in a position of having to assess the relative needs of one patient over another altogether, being forced to make value judgements that may require the aggregation of one person's welfare over another in situations where duties may have to be compromised in favour of the greater good principle. Such scenarios clearly bring in other ethical principles of justice and fairness. The whole area of the study of ethics is exciting and demands that we examine closely our decision-making processes in often complex ethical dilemmas if we are to ensure that the actions we take are right actions for all concerned. Further study of the ethics of health care is recommended.

Responsibility and accountability in law

There are three main areas of law concerned with health care practice:

- criminal law, for example illegal abortion and the illegal prescribing of drugs
- tort, which provides for compensation in cases of malpractice or negligence
- family law, which deals with issues relating to parenthood, surrogacy, parental rights and so on.

There is one further area, that of contract law, which may be used in private medicine where it is felt that there has been a breach of contract. In general, health care law basically centres around issues of negligence, consent, confidentiality and drug-induced injuries.

As in all other areas of law, it is the evolvement of case law that determines how legal issues in health care will be dealt with. The emergence of the individual nurse practitioner and the *Scope of Professional Practice* (UKCC 1992b) have required nurses to look more closely at case law related to health care matters as it has been developed and applied in medicine.

Negligence

In order to pursue a case of negligence against a health care professional, there is a need first of all to prove that there was a duty to care that was breached in some way as to cause harm warranting damages. A duty to care is defined thus:

> If a person holds himself as possessing a special skill and knowledge by or on behalf of a patient, he owes a duty to that patient to use due caution in undertaking the treatment.
>
> (R v. Bateman, cited in Kennedy and Grubb 1994, p. 400)

Any health care professional who undertakes the care of a patient in the NHS or privately owes the patient the common law duty to care. Once accepted as a patient, the above duty to care applies, and failure to treat is as actionable as any harm caused by negligent action.

Once that duty to care is established, there is a need further to ensure good professional practice. In determining negligence in medical treatment, the patient would then have to prove that the standard of care or treatment fell below that expected by the law and that there was therefore fault in a legal sense.

Good standards of practice were established in Bolam v. Friern Hospital Management Committee 1957 and now constitute what is known as the 'professional standards practice'; in essence:

> The test is the standard of the ordinary skilled man exercising or professing to have that special skill. A man need not possess the highest expert skill at the risk of being found negligent. It is a well-established law that it is sufficient if he exercises the ordinary skill of an ordinary man exercising that particular art.
>
> (Mason and McCall Smith 1994, p. 199)

Nevertheless he is professing a particular skill and should have the degree of competence and standards set by the ordinary skilful practitioner and expected by his profession.

When applied to nursing, this means that the test for the standard of care, that is, exercising the ordinary skill of an ordinary competent person within that speciality, can be equally applied. In order to prove negligence in nursing, there is a need to prove that the nurse acted contrary to good standards of practice. There are clear implications here for nurses who prescribe, that is, the need to be conversant with the NPF, the indications and contraindications of medications and products, their side-effects and the correct safe methods of administration. Perhaps most important of all is the need for good sound assessment skills before issuing a prescription.

In English law, then, the nurse is unlikely to be held liable in negligence if she acts in accordance with standard professional practice. However, Fletcher *et al.* (1995) question whether such obedience to rules could stifle the individual practice so implicit within the *Scope of Professional Practice* (UKCC 1992b). They suggest that, providing the nurse can use research-based evidence to justify her approach and actions, the patient would be unlikely to succeed in his complaint.

Nurse liability in prescribing

The basic common law principle is that an employer is liable for the negligent acts or omissions committed by his employee in the course of his employment. This is known as vicarious liability (Korgaonker and Tribe 1995). Employers are insured to cover their vicarious liability for employees' actions. Applied to nurse prescribing, the Crown Report (DoH 1989) states:

> We have also considered the issue of legal liability for nurse prescribers. Our understanding is this should not give rise to any new principle since, where a nurse undertakes prescribing as part of her normal duties of employment, the Health Authority as her employer is vicariously liable for her actions. Such vicarious liability extends to claims for damages against staff arising from alleged negligence in the performance of official duties. Most nurses obtain additional professional indemnity by means of their membership of a professional organisation or trade union.
>
> (p. 57)

However, this does not completely relieve the employee of any liability to the patient or client, who may well seek compensation from both employer and employee.

There are clearly strict guidelines governing the prescribing and administration of medicines in order to protect the public, and local protocols should reflect these guidelines. It would, however, be prudent for the nurse prescriber to ensure that local policy and protocols do not compromise or conflict with NHS Executive guidelines (1997) or their professional Code of Conduct.

Consent

In medical treatment, any non-consensual touching of the patient is essentially classed as battery in law. While such actions are very rarely pursued, there has been much litigation in the past decade relating to issues of consent, particularly informed consent. As far as consent to treatment is concerned, a patient has a right under common law to give or withhold consent prior to examination or treatment, the maxim being:

> every human being of adult years and sound mind has a right to determine what shall be done with his own body.
> (cited in Mason and McCall Smith 1994, p. 219)

Such consent to treatment or procedure should be obtained by the person who is to carry it out. For that consent to be valid, it should ideally be free, rational and informed, that is, all possible known risks and alternatives should be explored and pointed out to the patient so that he or she can make a balanced judgement on whether to accept the treatment or care offered:

> Work in an open and co-operative manner with patients, clients and their families, foster their independence and recognise and respect their involvement in the planning and delivery of care.
> (UKCC 1992a, cl. 5)

If a patient is not given sufficient information regarding proposed treatment and suffers in some way as a result, he may pursue a case of negligence against the health care professional, on the basis that, had he been given full information and explanation, he would probably have refused such care or treatment.

Great care is therefore needed by the nurse prescriber to ensure that all relevant information about proposed treatment, including any adverse effects, is given to the patient to ensure that full informed consent has taken place. The paternalist might argue that there may be situations in which treatment is justified even when the patient might object, on the basis that the proposed treatment is in the patient's best interests. There are certain narrowly defined legal justifications for proceeding without consent, which relate mainly to the unconscious or incompetent patient, or urgent situations where consent is not possible.

The UKCC *Guidelines for Professional Practice* (1996) have this to say about consent:

> It is important that the person proposing to perform a procedure should obtain consent, although there may be some urgent situations where another practitioner can do so.
>
> (cl. 29)

Although this statement relates to consent in general terms it can be quite easily related to nurse prescribing. It goes further, suggesting that the nurse is often best placed to know the emotions, views and concerns of the patient. This is particularly pertinent in the community setting, where strong interpersonal relationships may develop between nurse, patient and family, often over long periods of time.

These guidelines also deal with issues of truthfulness and state quite clearly that giving patients and clients information empowers them, and that to deny choice by insufficient or inaccurate information is to deny them their rights and thus diminish their dignity and independence (UKCC 1996). It would clearly be extremely difficult to uphold one of the prima-facie principles of health care ethics, that of autonomy, if patients did not have the necessary information to make informed choices.

In the treatment of children under 16 years, parental consent is essential where it is considered that the child does not have sufficient understanding to consent for himself, as in the 'Gillick competence' test (Mason and McCall Smith 1994). This is a particularly complex legal ruling that essentially endorsed the rights of 'competent minors' to consent to their own medical care and treatment in certain circumstances, that is, that they have sufficient understanding to fully appreciate the proposed treatment and all that it entails. These are features borne out in the fundamental principles of the Children Act 1989.

Generally, however, parental consent should be sought for the under-16-year-olds. There are two exceptions:

1. where it is clearly in the child's best interests
2. when it would result in an unacceptable delay of essential treatment.

Such situations may well not be those met frequently by the nurse prescriber, but there could be instances relating to the prescribing of topical applications, for example head infestation treatments or wound applications, that might require the nurse to take the child's views into account. The onus for assessing the competence of minors in terms of their ability to consent to treatment lies very much with the health care professional involved.

Product liability

Product liability is part of the Consumer Protection Act 1987. However, a producer may escape liability if it can be shown that the equipment was not used or maintained in accordance with the instructions or if medications are not stored in accordance with the recommendations. Therefore care needs to be exercised when equipment such as nebulisers is used or when vaccines and topical applications need to be stored.

Conclusion

As the role of the nurse continues to develop and increase with advances in medical science and technology, and wider issues such as the current political climate that calls for a reduction in junior doctors' hours, placing more responsibility on the nurse, nurses must continue to be guided by the *Code of Professional Conduct* (UKCC 1992a) and the *Scope of Professional Practice* (UKCC 1992b). Both these documents stress the importance of maintaining professional knowledge and competence, and emphasise the personal responsibility and accountability for practice. Any nurse who undertakes a task for which she is not trained or competent may be held accountable to her professional body; if the patient suffers harm, the nurse may be liable for negligence and held to account by the law, her profession or both. It is thus vital that all nurses engaging in nurse prescribing do not simply complete the necessary course but are able to take on board all the ongoing responsibilities that go with their new role.

References

Beauchamp, T.L. and Childress, J.F. (1994) *Principles of Biomedical Ethics*, 4th edn. Oxford University Press, Oxford.

Brown, J.M., Kitson, A.L. and McKnight T.J. (1992) *Challenges in Caring*. Chapman & Hall, London.

Dock, S. (1917) The relation of the nurse to the doctor and the doctor to the nurse. *American Journal of Nursing* 17: 394.

DoH (1989) *Report of the Advisory Group on Nurse Prescribing* (Crown Report). HMSO, London.

DoH (1992) *The Patient's Charter.* HMSO, London.

ENB (1994) *Nurse Prescribing. Open Learning Pack*. ENB, London.

Fletcher, N., Holt, J., Brazier M. and Harris, J. (1995) *Ethics Law and Nursing*. Manchester University Press, Manchester.

Grubb, I. and Kennedy, A. (1994) *Medical Law*, 2nd edn. Butterworth, London.

Korgaonker, G. and Tribe, D. (1995) *Law for Nurses*. Cavendish Publishing, London.

Koehn, D. (1994) *The Groundwork of Professional Ethics*. Routledge, London.

Mason, J.K. and McCall Smith, R.A. (1994) *Law and Medical Ethics,* 4th edn. Butterworth, London.

NHS Executive HQ (1997) *Nurse Prescribing Guidance*, *April* NHS, Leeds.

Tadd, V. (1994) Professional codes: an exercise in tokenism. *Nursing Ethics* 1(1): 15-23.

Thompson, I.E., Melia, K.M. and Boyd, K.M. (1994) *Nursing Ethics*. Churchill Livingstone, Edinburgh.

UKCC (1992a) *Code of Professional Conduct*. UKCC, London.

UKCC (1992b) *Scope of Professional Practice*. UKCC, London.

UKCC (1992c) *Standards for the Administration of Medicines*. UKCC, London.

UKCC (1993) *Standards for Records and Record Keeping*. UKCC, London.

UKCC (1996) *Guidelines for Professional Practice*. UKCC, London.

3 Assessment and evaluation in nurse prescribing

Jennifer Humphries

The focus of this chapter is to consider some of the principles of assessment and evaluation in the nursing care of patients and clients. Nurse prescribing has the potential to allow community practitioners to contemplate their assessment and evaluation approaches, and the chapter will examine some theoretical perspectives and consider how these apply when nurses are prescribers. The section will also look at the practical factors associated with assessment and evaluation specifically related to nurse prescribing in the community.

Assessment

The assessment of patients and clients often involves the collection of large amounts of information that the specialist community practitioner uses to determine health status and needs, and to plan appropriate care. Nurse prescribers use the same skills and strategies as used prior to qualification, but the assessment now has the added dimension of a possible nurse prescription. In some circumstances, the nurse or health visitor will be able to anticipate a prescribing episode; for example, a practice nurse undertaking vaccinations may routinely write a prescription for paracetamol to reduce post-immunisation pyrexia. Other prescribing may depend upon the features that arise during an encounter and will result in a prescription being generated immediately, for example a health visitor prescribing clotrimazole for an infant with nappy-area thrush. A third type of prescribing incident is a combination of the first two. In this situation, the nurse or health visitor has previously given care or offered advice and is returning to reassess, with the anticipation of prescribing if the original programme or strategy has been unsuccessful. For example, a district nurse may provide dietary advice for constipation and later prescribe a laxative.

The question, then, is whether prescribing becomes paramount in the patient/client assessment. The short answer is, of course not. A community nurse does not cease being a health visitor, practice nurse or district nurse when she becomes a prescriber, and, for many current prescribers, writing a prescription remains a rare event. Assessment of the patient or client is as before, but, should certain types of treatment included in the NPF be required, the nurse or health visitor is able to supply them by writing a prescription.

Models of care

In assessing patients and clients, nurses adopt a method of collecting and organising the information to plan and implement care. A variety of models are available to assist the practitioner in determining patient/client health status, identifying problems or needs and making decisions about the care delivery. Cormack and Reynolds (1992) describe a model as:

> a statement which causes nurses to perceive patients, their environment and their health/illness status in a specific way. It influences the way in which nurses understand and interpret the aetiology of pathology and of nursing needs, how these needs are identified, and how appropriate nursing intervention is selected to meet those needs, and the subsequent evaluation of that intervention.
>
> (p. 1473)

Some models are developed specifically for use by nurses, while others have been adapted from, for example, psychology or health promotion. Most models currently used by community practitioners, whether of nursing or borrowed from another discipline, are likely to be suitable for nurse prescribing. However, nurse prescribing is a new realm of nursing practice and affords practitioners the ideal opportunity for appraising existing frameworks or models used in current practice.

Sbaih (1997) suggests that a framework for care for use by community nurses should provide:

- a common starting place for nurses and clients
- a guide for the development of questions by the nurse, client and family to gain information
- a basis for participation and collaboration
- an opportunity for reflection on care-giving.

These points are useful for nurse prescribers who wish critically to evaluate the pertinence of a current model for nurse prescribing or to consider the suitability of a new approach.

Nursing knowledge and skills in assessing patients and clients

It is evident that a diagnosis has to have been reached in order to prescribe. Some nurses may initially feel uncomfortable with this since diagnosing has traditionally been the domain of doctors. Further examination, however, shows that diagnosis is not necessarily a daunting prospect. Consider first that nursing diagnosis is well established and forms the basis of episodes of care. Nurses have the skills to assess, plan, implement and subsequently evaluate nursing intervention.

Second, nursing intervention, whether in the community or hospital, frequently involves giving advice about prescribed medication. In the community setting, following assessment, nurses often advise clients and patients about over-the-counter preparations. A survey by *Community Nurse* magazine (Anderson 1995) found that 73 per cent of practice nurse respondents were involved in a clinic where they influenced changes of patients' medication, and 93 per cent of health visitor respondents regularly gave advice about over-the-counter medication. Advice about medication is sometimes little more than providing the name of a product, but it often involves detailed information about the use, effects and storage of the drug. Clearly, this is health education; it is advice based on a theoretical and practical knowledge of the preparation and on professional experience of product use by other patients and clients.

Third, nurses are always accountable for their practice; prescribing does not make a nurse more accountable. Prescribing, rather than advising on a product, may be less risky for both nurse and patient. The nurse prescriber may ultimately have more, rather than less, control over the episode of care, and the patient or client will arguably receive more comprehensive information about a nurse-prescribed product in the context of the whole assessment process than if he or she went to the pharmacist. The likelihood of fragmented care is reduced, and the patient may feel that a prescribed item is of more value than one bought from the pharmacy.

Finally, the diagnosis of conditions within community nursing practice is not new; indeed, when nurse prescribing was first advocated, it was noted that district nurses were requesting prescriptions for some products to treat certain conditions (DHSS 1986). Health visitors too have often asked GPs to write a prescription for a specific preparation to treat an infant's oral thrush or nappy rash. So nurses are diagnosing. Assessing patients and clients often results in a medical diagnosis that, before nurse prescribing, meant that the planning and implementation of patient care included a referral to the GP. The change when viewed in this context may appear less dramatic, the assessment of the same patient or client resulting in the same diagnosis, but the nursing intervention now being one of prescribing rather than referral. The government specifically acknowledges the skills of nurses in some diagnoses, the recent White Paper (DoH 1997) advocating an NHS helpline staffed by nurses, from which members of the public are able to seek information and advice about health and medical conditions. Here, a level of medical diagnosis is required.

If nurses and health visitors are to prescribe, they clearly have to be competent to do so. The training is important, and most practitioners will feel suitably equipped to prescribe in their role following this. However, in spite of the limited range of medications and treatments in the NPF, there may be those practitioners who do not feel sufficiently skilled to prescribe certain preparations. Clearly, the more experience a professional has in dealing with a condition, the more confident he or she is likely to feel about prescribing treatment for that condition. For example, some nurses and health visitors may have extensive and up-to-date knowledge of scabies, while others may have had little experience of the condition. A district nurse being alerted to head lice in a home for the care of elderly people may prefer to refer to her practice nurse or health visitor colleagues even though she can legally prescribe appropriate lotions. It may be only when a situation arises that nurses and health visitors become aware of a lack of recent experience having reduced their confidence in their diagnosis and treatment of a condition. The obvious solution in the immediate situation is to refer to a colleague who does feel competent, be it to another nurse or the GP, but in the longer term it can be something of which a nurse prescriber may feel compelled to gain additional knowledge and experience. Much will depend on the context in which the professional works, and the community or practice profile can serve as a useful method of determining the needs of the population relating specifically to prescribing. Assessing the needs of communities may establish the prevalence of head lice or other conditions, and a current lack of knowledge of these conditions would prevent nurse prescribers from fulfilling not just their prescribing role, but also a public health function. Practitioners have a professional responsibility to ensure competence before prescribing, and the presentation of clearly defined information can serve as a tool to ask for additional training. Updating on aspects of pharmacology may be required before a nurse feels competent to prescribe some of the preparations in the NPF (Courtney and Butler 1998).

Community and practice profiling may prove useful in relation to prescribing assessment. Apart from the obvious collection of prescription analysis and cost (PACT) data that clearly demonstrate prescribing allocation, nurses and health visitors may be able to determine particular places where health education strategies could prove useful. For example, a community-wide programme offering dietary advice may result in fewer requests for prescriptions for laxatives. A local initiative promoting healthy skin and good examples of skin care may result in more nurse prescriptions for emollients in the short term. However, in the longer term, the outcome for patients with dry skin conditions is likely to improve.

All community nurses use their knowledge and skills in assessing patients and regularly make decisions about the need for patients or clients to consult a doctor. A prescribing practitioner maintains this option. The ability to prescribe does not mean that it will always be the intervention of choice. Most practitioners therefore will continue to use their skills to identify and define the patients' complaints and discriminate these from other possible conditions. As always, referral to a medical colleague for evaluation and possible treatment continues to be one alternative.

Clinical decision-making

Prescribing assessment is part of the whole assessment procedure, but, for some new prescribers, the use of skills and knowledge in making the clinical decision may become explicit, being a conscious decision to use the knowledge and practise the skills. Luker and Kenrick (1992) examined the sources of influence on the clinical decisions of community nurses in the context of nurse prescribing. The results of the small exploratory study undertaken before the nurse prescribing pilot indicated that even highly skilled practitioners were often unable to articulate the source of their knowledge for clinical decisions. This is not a new phenomenon, Benner (1994) suggesting that expert practitioners regard situations holistically, drawing on experiences and being unconsciously guided by intuition and 'gut feelings'. Luker and Kenrick (1992) acknowledge that experiential knowledge may be scientific knowledge that has been integrated by the practitioner and reclassified. These authors do not devalue clinical experience, although they do suggest that it may be used at the expense of science. Moreover, they note that it is nurses' lack of ability to articulate the source of their knowledge that may impede their credibility and inhibit the transmission of the knowledge to new practitioners. Peate's (1996) small investigation into how nurses make decisions about patient medication concluded that nurses use a variety of reasons, often dependent on context. Schober (1993) notes the relationship between nursing theory and nursing knowledge:

> Nursing is essentially a practice discipline, but the quality of practice depends upon attitudes, knowledge and abilities for effective care. The way nurses use knowledge and apply theory will influence their approach to nursing; sound decision making depends upon using knowledge expertly.
>
> (p. 310)

Prescribing is just one way of providing nursing care, the decision to prescribe being ultimately the nurse's. Brew (1997 p. 239) reminds us that nurses need to be professionally and legally accountable for their actions and offers the following factors for consideration concerning nurse prescribing:

- The patient's circumstances, including current medication
- The patient's past medical history
- The patient's current and anticipated health status
- Thorough knowledge of the item to be prescribed, its therapeutic action, side effects, dosage and interaction
- Thorough knowledge of alternatives to prescribing
- Frequency of use in a variety of circumstances.

Assessment allows the nurse to establish whether prescribing is the most appropriate intervention. Once this decision has been reached, the assessment process continues within the context of prescribing. To ensure safe and effective prescribing, it is vital to assess current medication or treatment in order to guard against possible drug interactions. A variety of strategies may need to be employed to find out the information. People do not necessarily perceive medication bought from a supermarket as a drug and may offer information only about prescribed items. Asking to see products enables the nurse to determine the ingredients contained in some proprietary brands and affords an opportunity for health education, including discussing the storage and use of medicines and stressing the importance of using prescribed products only for the person named on the prescription and not for family or friends.

Determining previous medication and treatment is also essential since efficacy in the past can be significant in deciding specific products. Although the NPF is currently quite limited, it does contain alternatives, for example the option of miconazole or nystatin for oral thrush, and the option of soluble paracetamol for those who have difficulty swallowing tablets. There is also a reasonable range of laxatives in the NPF, and the choice of wound dressings for nurse prescribers is extensive. Whenever possible, nurses should involve patients in decisions about care, and prescribing is no different in this. Including patients or clients in assessing their health status and needs may be influential in encouraging compliance with the treatment prescribed.

Evaluation

Evaluating the quality of health care is essential for all health professionals. The concept is not new: McIntyre (1995) cites Florence Nightingale as advocating the systematic collection of information to improve patient treatment. Various terms are used when discussing evaluation in health care, including 'clinical audit', 'quality initiatives' and 'measuring effectiveness'. Luker (1992) notes that evaluation is often referred to by other terms, for example 'appraisal' or 'assessment'. Many of the principles apply to the whole range of evaluation strategies. Essentially, the idea of nursing evaluation is to determine whether nursing intervention has been effective. If it has, it allows the principles employed to be repeated for the benefit of other patients and clients, and allows examples of good practice to be passed on to other practitioners so that their patients and clients can also profit. The evaluation of an activity shown not to be satisfactory prevents its repetition, and therefore this too ultimately results in improved patient care.

Evaluation is part of the nursing process and constitutes a cyclical activity. It is not always straightforward: some aspects of evaluation are informal, and there may be difficulty in isolating particular issues for evaluation since they may not be readily delineated from other parts of the care provided. An issue of particular relevance to community nursing is the often long-term nature of intervention, the impact not becoming apparent for months or years; even then, as a health promotion or disease prevention intervention, it can be difficult to measure. An independent prescribing activity, however, often offers community nurses the opportunity for a more accelerated evaluation.

The evaluation of nursing intervention can range from the simple to the highly complex depending on what is being evaluated, and it is this point that is perhaps the crux of any evaluation scheme. It is essential to determine exactly what is being evaluated and to decide appropriate methods of collecting and analysing the information that will address the evaluation plan.

One manner of describing the mechanisms associated with evaluation is to divide the whole into three distinct arenas: structure, process and outcome (Donabedian 1980). In nurse prescribing, examples of structure would be the composition of the teams providing the prescribing care and the expertise of the staff. The process would be the delivery of the prescribing care, and the outcome would be the effectiveness of that care.

Structure

The main facets for structure of evaluation are likely to bring to the fore the expertise of the nurse who prescribes. This is an interesting concept because the impetus behind nurse prescribing came from the premise that community nurses had the expertise and were, in many cases, prescribing informally (DHSS 1986). Nevertheless, since the notion of nurses taking on the role formally was first documented, there have been reservations about the knowledge and expertise that community nurses possess. Even before the original pilot programme began, a study by While and Rees (1993) suggested that the knowledge base for prescribing among district nurses and health visitors was restricted. Although this is an acknowledged small-scale study using a convenience sample of nurses and health visitors, the lack of knowledge of conditions and the products intended to treat them was remarkable. These nurses were not prescribers, and, while this does not excuse the poor knowledge base, it should also be noted that most of the subjects in While and Rees's study recognised the need for further training. Luker *et al.*'s (1997a) evaluation of the nurse prescribing pilot suggests that the content of the nurse prescribers' training course was good and adequately prepared the nurses for their role as prescribers. It has to be considered that just because nurses can prescribe, this does not mean that they will, and the prescribing nurses' view is that they would only prescribe if they had the necessary training and experience (Luker *et al.* 1997b).

Process

Within the episode of patient or client care, the evaluations of nursing activity and patient outcome are frequently integrated. For example, the effectiveness of a prescription for paracetamol (the outcome) can usually be determined very rapidly, but the prescription will not have been issued in isolation, and it is therefore vital that process evaluation is incorporated. The parents of a baby with post-immunisation pyrexia will also have been given advice about the care of the infant concerning clothing, tepid sponging and handling. A patient with mild-to-moderate pain will have been given additional information about management that addresses the source of the pain. In both instances, the patient or client will have been told what to do if the problem persists in spite of the medication.

Thus the information supplied with the prescription is a vital aspect of the role of the nurse prescriber, since incorrect usage can result in the treatment being ineffective. Patients and clients require clear and concise information about the items prescribed; they should be told about the effects of the medication or treatment and how soon these may be expected. Some preparations have side-effects, and, although most are rare and/or mild, information about these can assist patients in discriminating between these and a severe adverse reaction and can help to ensure that the treatment is not stopped prematurely. Clear instructions about when and how to take the medication, any special precautions and what to do if they have any concerns should be given verbally and, if necessary, in written form.

Outcome

Outcome evaluation may initially seem to be the most obvious form of evaluation for nurse prescribers. Was the prescription effective? Has the headache gone, the constipation resolved, the wound healed, the thrush cleared? Its appeal is evident because what health professionals ultimately want to know is what the results of the intervention were for the patient; according to McIntyre (1995), many would consider outcome to be the most relevant indicator of quality of care.

Despite its immediate appeal, outcome evaluation can be complex to measure. Patient outcome is notoriously difficult to link to, or separate from, clinical (nursing or medical) intervention. Remember the old adage 'the operation was a success but the patient died'. This problem is compounded by the nature of community nursing, because, unlike in a hospital setting where care is provided on a 24-hour basis, hands-on or face-to-face contact occupies a very small part of the care package. So many other factors impinge on the intervention that it is very difficult to ascertain how far the outcome relates to the process. The complexity of an apparently simple intervention is not confined to nurse prescribers, so prescribing nurses are not subjected to new dilemmas about appropriate ways of evaluating nursing intervention and the link to patient outcome. However, nurse prescribing can add a slightly different dimension. Non-prescribing community nurses do offer advice about medication for pyrexia and pain, recommending paracetamol from the pharmacy or often from the home medicine cabinet, so evaluation of the intervention is thus already part of the care provided. A nurse prescriber, however, may evaluate the appropriateness of writing the prescription and, on reflection, may question whether the patient or client should have been advised to buy the product. Financial and social circumstances are likely to impinge on the decision to prescribe (Luker *et al.* 1997a), and a review could result in alterations to existing practice.

Patient/client satisfaction

When attempting to evaluate effectiveness, it is imperative to decide not only what to evaluate, but also whose judgement is to be used. In the area of nurse prescribing, it is possible that the nurse/health visitor and patient/client may view the situation differently. Take, for example, the patient with a leg wound who would have preferred a different dressing despite the rational and careful explanation by the district nurse, or the mother of a constipated toddler who views the detailed health education given by the health visitor as being of less use than a prescription for a laxative. Consider too the patient of a practice nurse who wanted a prescription for the treatment of vaginal thrush and was disappointed to know that it was not available on a nurse prescription. Patient satisfaction is important, and some nurse prescribers may choose to modify their treatment if they consider that the patient is more likely to comply and/or has great faith in the product, especially if there is no or little difference between the two treatments. There are undoubtedly those patients and clients who have ultimate faith in professional expertise; many community nurses and health visitors know of individuals and families who would not go to the pharmacy for an over-the-counter preparation but who would adhere rigorously to the instructions that accompany a prescription. Professional judgement is part of a nurse's role, and the decision to prescribe rests with the prescriber. The crucial aspect is whether the prescriber has a rational justification for the decision.

Clinical audit

Clinical audit is a formal and systematic analysis of practice that includes aspects of the quality of care provided, procedures, the use of resources and the resulting outcome. Audit is an ideal procedure for use with nurse prescribing because it enables the prescribing to be analysed objectively as a specific area of practice.

Another advantage of audit for nurse prescribing is that it frequently involves standard-setting whereby specific and measurable criteria are identified for detailed examination. Ideally, the standard should be agreed by all staff who are to participate in the audit. Setting standards is often based on previous research, and, in this, nurse prescribers will initially have little British nurse prescribing evidence of practice to which to refer. This should not deter nurse prescribers from attempting audit from the outset since evidence of good practice is an acceptable alternative. The importance of keeping up to date with developments in nursing is essential. Information about research and practice that may be applicable in the field of nurse prescribing can be found in national and international nursing journals and obtained from professional nursing bodies. A critical analysis of the prescribing activity of other professional groups, such as GPs, may prove useful to nurse prescribers. This information may be gained informally from GP colleagues who are willing to share their personal experiences or from medical publications.

Although nurse prescribing in other countries may not be directly transferable to British experience, useful comparisons may be made to develop prescribing practice. Shepherd et al. (1996) note that American studies on nurse prescribing suggest that financial savings on administrative overheads have been made. They also note that, in Australia, nurses have been particularly active in developing policy in the quality use of medicines. Comparing prescribing practice with agreed standards should also identify other issues for audit and allow the cycle to begin again.

Clinical supervision

One of the recommendations of the evaluation of nurse prescribing is that a model of clinical supervision is necessary to ensure the development of effective nursing practice (Luker *et al.* 1997a).

Swain (1995) suggests that clinical supervision is now an established aspect of professional development for nurses, midwives and health visitors. The idea of clinical supervision in caring for patients and clients is not new, although permeation of the principle received considerable impetus through *A Vision for the Future* (NHSME 1993). Clinical supervision is described in this document as:

> a term used to describe a formal process of professional support and learning which enables individual practitioners to develop knowledge and competence, assume responsibility for their own practice and enhance consumer protection and the safety of care in complex clinical situations. It is central to the process of learning and to the expansion of the scope of practice and should be seen as a means of encouraging self assessment and analytical and reflective skills.

> (p. 15)

The intention of clinical supervision is therefore to enable practitioners to reflect on practice in a creative and supportive environment, allowing an opportunity for learning and professional development. Clinical supervision is also about ensuring high-quality care for patients and clients. Although Butterworth *et al.* (1997) suggest that there are a number of devotees of clinical supervision among British nurses, they acknowledge that the impact on patient care and the benefits for professionals are not well demonstrated by research.

As nurse prescribing is a new venture, the processes involved in clinical supervision should be documented in order to enable subsequent prescribers to benefit. Some community nurses and health visitors may feel that the change of status to nurse prescriber is barely noticeable, that the ability to prescribe is simply a legitimisation of existing practice anyway. However, anecdotal evidence from nurse prescribing students is supported by the findings of the evaluation study (Luker *et al.* 1997a) that new prescribers are highly aware of their new role. There are bound to be some uncertainties for newly qualified prescribers, and advice and support are essential. While the anxiety about writing prescriptions may be short lived, it should not be belittled, and clinical supervision can provide practitioners with a way of working through the anxieties so that confidence in clinical practice and prescribing can develop.

Evaluating personal development

Nurses are increasingly being confronted with a variety of strategies that assist them to evaluate their own clinical expertise and professional development. The mandatory requirement from the UKCC (1997) obliges every nurse, midwife and health visitor to keep an up-to-date profile of his or her professional development. As well as being a record of learning and achievement, the profile can be useful in encouraging practitioners to reflect on their experiences and can also help to link theory and practice. For some, the training to become a nurse prescriber may be the first formal undertaking of study for some time. It can provide a catalyst for the reflection of current practice and encourage an elaboration of the processes of reflection to encompass prescribing. Nurse prescribers may find other methods of encouraging reflection useful, for example describing experiences to colleagues and peers, as in case presentations or significant incident discussions in both formal and informal situations. Both the open learning pack (ENB 1994) and the taught programme encourage prescribers to assess their own progress in prescribing, and it is crucial that nurse prescribers constantly review their expertise and competence. Existing local practices and policies can allow the incorporation of prescribing evaluation, for example community nursing team meetings, managerial meetings, individual performance review, primary health care team meetings and local meetings of professional associations.

Scope of Professional Practice

The intention of the *Scope of Professional Practice* (UKCC 1992) is to encourage nurses to develop their skills and expertise in relation to their own situation, for example their clinical area, and their decision to learn is to meet the needs of patients or clients within that area. Interestingly, the *Scope of Professional Practice* deliberately rejected the need for additional certification that would enable practitioners to extend their roles; instead, 'role expansion' was the favoured term because it emphasised the practitioners' own decision to learn and reflected their own situation. Nurse prescribing would appear to fit more comfortably with the extended role definition. As Land *et al.* (1996) note, extended roles involve undertaking new tasks that frequently require technical skills likely to have come from other groups. Moreover, the only way in which nurses can become prescribers is by way of the qualification that is gained by completing an approved course and passing an examination. However, the certificate, as with any other professional nursing qualification, does not remove the nurse's own responsibility for competent practice. Instead it adds a further dimension to existing practice and compels nurse prescribers to recognise their own level of competence and decline duties for which they do not feel prepared. This is not an unusual phenomenon in prescribing. A GP from the evaluation study by Luker *et al.* (1997b) noted that, although he had the potential to prescribe from the whole of the *British National Formulary* (BNF), he clearly would not do so if he did not feel competent. He continues regarding nurse prescribing, 'I am aware that this system is already operative because the health visitors do not prescribe dressing packs because it is not within their sphere of work' (p. 37). The *Scope of Professional Practice* (UKCC 1992) should allow nurse prescribers to evaluate their expertise in prescribing in the context of their own area, caseload and the products currently available in the NPF.

Documentation

Wyatt (1995) argues the importance of high-quality data in both research and audit. Nurse prescribers have to ensure accurate recording of their prescribing, so it has great potential in the area of audit and for future research studies about prescribing. Toms (1992) proposes that 'district nurses often look upon recording information as a secondary procedure to actually giving care, placing little value and emphasis on it' (p. 1490). She goes on to suggest that accurate documentation is essential and can provide an encouraging record of nursing skills. Luker (1992) supports this view, stating that 'the only area of a community health nurse's work which can readily be monitored is her record keeping' (p. 186). Nurse prescribers need also to provide details of the information given to the patient concerning management of the condition and the product prescribed. In some cases, a nurse may make the decision not to prescribe, perhaps advising a GP consultation or an over-the-counter preparation; documentation can allow the nurse to audit his or her prescribing decisions and offers a useful impetus for personal professional reflection.

Conclusion

This chapter has considered the skills and expertise of the specialist community practitioner who is assessing and evaluating patient care in the context of nurse prescribing. Various strategies and ideas have been put forward that illustrate the essential sameness to practise without the ability to prescribe, while also recognising the potential evolution that nurse prescribing presents for the review and development of practice.

References

Anderson, P. (1995) Your role in prescribing. *Community Nurse* 1(11): 20–2.
Benner, P. (1984) *From Novice to Expert: Excellence and Power in Clinical Nursing Practice*. Addison-Wesley, Reading, MA.
Brew, M. (1997) Nurse prescribing. In Burley, S., Mitchell, E.E., Melling, K., Smith, M., Chilton, S. and Crumplin, C. (eds) *Contemporary Community Nursing*, pp. 229–43. Edward Arnold, London.
Butterworth, T., Jeacock, J., Carson, J. and White, E. (1997) Clinical supervision: a hornet's nest or honey pot? *Nursing Times* 93(44): 27–9.

Cormack, D.F.S. and Reynolds, W. (1992) Criteria for evaluating the clinical and practical utility of models used by nurses. *Journal of Advanced Nursing* **17**: 1472–8.

Courtney, M. and Butler, M. (1998) Nurse prescribing – the knowledge base. *Nursing Times* **94**(1): 40–2.

DoH (1986) *Neighbourhood Nursing: A Focus for Care* (Cumberlege Report). HMSO, London.

DoH (1997) *The New NHS: Modern, Dependable.* Stationery Office, London.

Donabedian, A. (1980) *Explorations in Quality Assessment and Monitoring. Vol 1: The Definition of Quality and Approaches to its Assessment.* Health Administration Press, Ann Arbor, MI.

ENB (1994) *Nurse Prescribing. Open Learning Pack.* ENB, London.

Land, L., Ni Mhaolrunaigh, S. and Castledine, G. (1996) Extent and effectiveness of the *Scope of Professional Practice. Nursing Times* **92**(35): 32–5.

Luker, K. (1992) Evaluating practice. In Luker, K. and Orr, J. (eds) *Health Visiting. Towards Community Health Nursing*, pp. 159–90. Blackwell Scientific, Oxford.

Luker, K.A. and Kenrick, M. (1992) An exploratory study of the sources of influence on the clinical decisions of community nurses. *Journal of Advanced Nursing* **17**: 457–66.

Luker, K.A., Austin, L., Hogg, C. *et al.* (1997a) Evaluation of Nurse Prescribing Final Report: Executive Summary. Unpublished report.

Luker, K.A., Austin, L., Willock, J., Ferguson, B. and Smith, K. (1997b) Nurses' and GPs' views of the nurse prescribers formulary. *Nursing Standard* **11**(22): 33–8.

McIntyre, N. (1995) Evaluation in clinical practice: problems, precedents and principles. *Journal of Evaluation in Clinical Practice* **1**(1): 5–13.

NHS Management Executive (1993) *A Vision for the Future.* DoH, London.

Peate, I. (1996) How nurses make decisions regarding patient medication. *British Journal of Nursing* **5**(7): 417–18, 435–7.

Sbaih, L. (1997) Models of care. In Skidmore, D. (ed.) *Community Care: Initial Training and Beyond*, pp. 75–103. Edward Arnold, London.

Schober, J. (1993) Frameworks for nursing practice. In Hinchcliff, S.M., Norman, S.E. and Schober, J.E. (eds) *Nursing Practice and Health Care*, 2nd edn, pp. 300–27. Edward Arnold, London.

Shepherd, E., Rafferty, A.M. and James, V. (1996) Prescribing the boundaries of nursing practice: professional regulation and nurse prescribing. *NTResearch* **1**(6): 465–78.

Swain, G. (1995) *Clinical Supervision: The Principles and Process.* Health Visitors Association, London.

Toms, E.C. (1992) Evaluating the quality of patient care in district nursing. *Journal of Advanced Nursing* **17**: 1489–95.

UKCC (1992) *Scope of Professional Practice.* UKCC, London.

UKCC (1997) *PREP and You.* UKCC, London.

While, A.E. and Rees, K.L. (1993) The knowledge base of health visitors and district nurses regarding products in the proposed formulary for nurse prescription. *Journal of Advanced Nursing* **18**: 1573–7.

Wyatt, J. (1995) Acquisition and use of clinical data for audit and research. Evaluation in clinical practice: problems, precedents and principles. *Journal of Evaluation in Clinical Practice* **1**(1): 15–27.

4 Responsibilities of prescribing

Rosalyn Anderson

Individual responsibilities as a prescriber

All prescribers have a personal and legal responsibility to ensure that the most appropriate items are selected to meet the needs of the patient in a safe and cost-effective manner. The legal responsibility for prescribing always lies with the person who signs the prescription. It is dangerous to prescribe on the recommendation of a third party (even another health professional) if the prescriber has not seen the patient. By considering cost in relation to not only product selection, but also quantities prescribed, the prescriber should demonstrate financial responsibility. This should only be considered after the needs of the patient have been identified, when selection between alternative products with a similar action, but different cost, may be an option. Cost should never be the primary consideration.

The prescriber has a responsibility to the pharmacist to ensure that intentions are precisely stated, not open to misinterpretation and, if hand-written, are perfectly legible. Although pharmacists have traditionally been expected to translate poorly written prescriptions, this is not acceptable and is fraught with dangers.

Security of prescriptions

Blank prescriptions should be regarded as blank cheques. Prescribers should never leave prescriptions unattended during a consultation. Prescriptions should be locked up when not in use and should not be left in a car.

Prescribers should always ensure that they use the appropriately preprinted prescription, with correct identifiers, to ensure that it is attributed and costed correctly. Practice nurse prescriptions are coloured differently from those of community nurses and health visitors, and each trust or practice is provided with individually identifiable prescriptions for all staff.

Prescription-writing requirements

For every professional involved in prescription-writing and interpretation, the safety of the patient is paramount. While there are legal requirements concerning the essential aspects of a prescription, there are additional recommendations to ensure that the pharmacist can accurately interpret the prescriber's wishes, check the doses prescribed, counsel patients appropriately and provide usable packs. If any information, such as age, is omitted, this process becomes more difficult and more time-consuming. Although age can be checked with the parent or guardian, other omissions may lead to considerable inconvenience for the patient if the prescriber has to be contacted by the pharmacist in order to clarify essential information. The following should be noted:

- A separate prescription must be written for each patient. In other words, nurses cannot prescribe a bulk pack of head lice lotion to treat a family.
- All prescriptions must be computer printed or written in ink.
- The prescriber must sign and date the prescriptions in ink.
- The prescriber must sign and date any alterations in ink.
- The age of children (and preferably of elderly patients too) must be stated.

Prescriptions must also include:

- the full name of the drug, dressing or appliance without the use of abbreviations, using the generic name where practicable. The brand name should be used for dressings and appliances to avoid the possibility of patients receiving an inappropriate product or even receiving a different product each time. Accurate patient medication records in pharmacies should help to identify previously issued products in order to update practice records

- the strength and relevant identifying factors, such as the sizes of dressings and catheters
- the dose and frequency where possible
- directions in English with no abbreviations
- the minimum dose intervals for drugs that can be taken only when needed, for example 'not more than every 6 hours'
- the quantity required, with consideration of the pack size.
- the quantities stated as follows:
  - less than 1 g: state in milligrams, for example 500 mg
  - more than 1 g: state in grams, for example 1.5 g
  - for liquids: state the strength per ml, for example 250 mg/ 5 ml
  ml, mg and g are acceptable abbreviations, but 'micrograms' should never be abbreviated.

Generic prescribing

As directed in the NPF, all products should, except where indicated otherwise, be prescribed by approved generic title as given in the formulary. This title is usually the chemical name of the product, as distinct from the brand names that manufacturers use to market their own particular versions of that generic product. Some products are available only from one manufacturer and are given a brand name, but the generic description should still be used. Other products are produced in branded and generic forms, while some are only produced as generics.

Many generic tablets or capsules are produced by the same manufacturer who produces the branded version or by a subsidiary of that company. In such cases, the product will be identical in every way to the branded product. Even when the generic manufacturer differs from the manufacturer of the brand, generic products now usually match the brand to avoid patient confusion. It is important for patients to be told that medicines will be generically prescribed, especially if they have previously received a branded product. There may be a more apparent difference between topical branded and generic products as the packaging may be markedly different. An example is Canesten cream, which patients may have received previously from the doctor, which is supplied in a tube and box differently coloured from those of the generic clotrimazole cream prescribed by nurses. Patients can be reassured that the contents of the tube contain exactly the same active ingredient and will treat the infection in the same way. Often, even when a generic product is prescribed, the patient will receive a branded product. This is because it is often cheaper for some pharmacists and wholesalers to purchase the brand rather than the generic product. However, in such cases, the prescriber is credited with prescribing generically, and the practice or trust is charged accordingly.

Both branded and generic products have to comply with the stringent licensing requirements of the Medicines Control Agency, and patients can be reassured that all are equally safe in terms of the manufacturing process and the quality of the final product.

Parallel imports

These are medicinal products that are produced and packaged elsewhere in the EEC and imported to the UK. The language of the exporting country is often apparent on the packaging, but none of the patient instructions should be in any language other than English. These products are often issued against generic prescriptions as, paradoxically, it is cheaper for the pharmacist to do this than to dispense a product manufactured and packaged in the UK. Patients can be reassured that these imported products must comply with the same high licensing standards that apply to products made in this country.

Additives or excipients in medicinal products or appliances

It is important to consider that certain patients may experience allergies to additives in medicines and other preparations. These components may differ between generic and branded products, and between appliances made by different manufacturers. A simple example is that some ointments and creams contain lanolin as a major emollient component, but this is for many patients a potent skin sensitiser. In terms of additives to improve flavouring, some medicines contain sugar and others do not. Where a sugar-free form is available, this should always be selected for children to reduce the risk of dental caries in those who receive regular medication. Such preparations are identified in the NPF.

Allergies to additives may become apparent when patients change to a generic product or even between brands, and between appliances such as catheters because of allergies to different plasticisers. While patients sometimes resist change from established products, the possibility of genuine allergy should not be ignored. If allergy is suspected, manufacturers should be asked for information on all the ingredients to enable the sensitising item to be identified and avoided in the future. Patients should be advised to carry information on any allergies, and notes and computer records should be clearly marked.

Influences on prescribing

All professionals with prescribing responsibility are subjected to external prescribing influences from advertisements, representatives, sponsored events, other professionals and even the public. Prescribers should ensure that they have adequate unbiased information to make prescribing decisions, without reference to any form of sponsored publication. They should also be aware of issues of relevance to the public, such as items under discussion in the media, in order to address public concerns or questions about items that they may prescribe. As prescribers generally are subject to great attention from pharmaceutical companies, nurse prescribers will be no exception. A practice policy should be drawn up in conjunction with all prescribers to detail the level of drug promotion that is acceptable, for example the number of sponsored meetings per month, and to agree an appointment system for pharmaceutical representatives in order to reduce frustrations on both sides.

Independent reference sources for prescribers

Easily accessible books

● *British National Formulary*
The BNF is jointly published every 6 months by the British

Medical Association and the Royal Pharmaceutical Society of Great Britain. It is a readily available reference source that includes all the medicinal products available for prescribing in the UK and also products restricted to hospital prescribing. It is important that a current edition is used as dosages and safety warnings may change. One example is that Lindane lotion and shampoo were included in the first NPF and deleted in January 1995 because of concerns about neurotoxicity in babies and infants. Appendix 8 of the BNF details urinary and stoma appliances and Appendix 9 shows wound management products. The NPF is included at the end of the BNF.

● *Drug Tariff*
This is published monthly by the DoH and gives prices and prescribing details, including pack sizes, for various nurse-prescribable products. Familiarity with this publication facilitates its usefulness, and the user should remember the following locations:

● generic oral and topical preparations (creams, ointments) – Part VIII
● wound management products – Part IXA
● catheters – Part IXA
● other incontinence appliances – Part IXB
● stoma appliances – Part IXC.

Other independent sources of prescribing information

Although the BNF gives some comparative therapeutic information, more detail will often be required in order to make a prescribing decision. Continuing education should facilitate rational, evidence-based prescribing and should enable prescribers to analyse critically research papers and pharmaceutical industry literature. Comparative information on drugs and other prescribable items can be resourced from local, regional and national drug information centres. Local pharmacists should be a useful starting point if information is required quickly. All general practices receive a regular drug information bulletin with separate editions for England (MeReC), Scotland (Medicines Resource) and Wales

(WeMeReC). This covers different therapeutic topics, with the emphasis on prescribing, and also usually includes comparative cost information. In Northern Ireland, the publication *Drug Data* is produced by the Regional Drug Information Service and covers similar topics. Nurse prescribers should ask to be added to appropriate mailing lists. From early 1999 MeReC will also produce a bulletin targeted specifically at nurse prescribers.

Drug and Therapeutics Bulletin

This is produced monthly by the publishers of *Which?*, the consumer magazine, but is written by health professionals for use by prescribers. It is particularly useful for reviews of new products in order to help prescribers to determine their place in the therapeutic armoury. Some issues cover reviews of drug groups, and a review of back issues is recommended.

Local drug information bulletins

Prescribers should check with local drug information centres (usually based in the pharmacy departments of the acute trusts) on the availability of local drug information bulletins. These may include comparative information on new drugs or may review the place of established products or therapies, especially where these are popular with local consultants. It may be possible to ask for a particular topic, for example recommendations for the management of infestations or the selection of wound management products, to be covered.

Primary care prescribing bulletins

These are usually produced by pharmaceutical and/or medical advisers in health authorities or commissions. They usually address current issues of relevance to primary care prescribing and to the primary–secondary care interface. They may report on local trends in GP and nurse prescribing.

Individual queries about prescribed items

These may be addressed to the local community pharmacist or local drug information centre. Specific information on incontinence appliances may be dealt with by the local continence adviser, while the specialist stoma nurse will answer queries concerning any stoma products. Both can help to determine suitable quantities to prescribe. It is important to remember that, in certain areas, these specialist posts are partially or totally sponsored, and postholders will therefore be most knowledgeable about the sponsoring company's products.

To prescribe or not?

This dilemma faces all prescribers many times throughout the day and is sometimes perceived as a way of ending a consultation. Such prescribing is often inappropriate, and patients may actually be more in need of time than a prescription.

Prescribers may also demonstrate suboptimal prescribing in the following ways:

- giving in to patient pressure to prescribe either an inappropriate drug and/or for an inappropriate reason, for example antibiotics for a probable viral infection
- repeating prescriptions for long periods of time with inadequate patient review (see below)
- prescribing new products without supporting clinical information to illustrate their advantages over existing products
- prescribing expensive products when equally effective cheaper products are readily available
- prescribing outdated products because of an inadequate updating of clinical knowledge.

The prescriber should therefore approach the prescribing process by adopting the following aims of good prescribing (Barber 1985) to:

- maximise effectiveness
- minimise risks
- minimise costs
- respect patient choices.

In order to meet these aims, the prescriber must consider many factors. The following list seems interminable but should become second nature as the good prescribing habit becomes established:

- Current and past medical problem – is a current diagnosis confirmed?
- The impact of other factors, such as smoking and alcohol intake, and diet.
- Over-the-counter medicines that the patient may be using.
- Currently prescribed drug therapy and indications for each prescribed item.
- Is a new prescription essential?
- Can any drugs or preparations be cancelled before adding new therapy?
- Are the safest and most effective products in use?
- Has cost been considered or are cheaper, equally safe and effective products available?
- Are drugs appropriate for the age of the patient in terms of not only dose, but also ease of application or administration?
- Can the patient take the drug correctly or apply it correctly?
- Has the patient suffered allergies in the past?
- Does the product contain potential allergens?
- Does the patient have any problems that may affect drug-handling in the body, for example renal or hepatic impairment, or pregnancy? See BNF: Appendix 2, Liver disease; Appendix 3, Renal impairment; Appendix 4, Pregnancy; Appendix 5, Breast-feeding; all of these contain useful guidance on drugs that may give problems in each circumstance and their probable clinical significance. Always refer any concerns to a doctor before prescribing.
- Are there any potential interactions between products? See BNF Appendix 1, Interactions, and check with the doctor if unsure.
- For how long should the treatment be needed?
- How often should the patient be reviewed in order to monitor the effectiveness of therapy?
- How will the response/improvement be measured?
- What is the correct description for the item required? This is particularly important for stoma and incontinence appliances.
- What is an appropriate quantity based on normal usage?

Prescribers must also be able to recognise personal limitations in order to enable appropriate referral to nursing or medical colleagues when the diagnosis is uncertain and the appropriate treatment unclear. When selecting products from the NPF, special attention should be paid to the clinical warning boxes, which make recommendations about the need to refer to a doctor for advice, for example before prescribing laxatives for children.

Cautions, contraindications, side-effects and adverse reactions

Cautions, contraindications and the prevention of adverse effects of therapy

Prescribers should aim to minimise the occurrence of adverse reactions to drug therapy by careful consideration of the need for additional medication. In detailing the points for consideration before prescribing additional treatments, various patient problems, for example renal and hepatic impairments, have been highlighted that can cause difficulties with certain drug treatments. Some drugs, particularly some systemic therapies, may be totally contraindicated in such patients, but always consult a doctor if there are concerns about any items in the NPF. BNF Appendix 2 (Liver disease) and Appendix 3 (Renal impairment) provide useful information on drugs to be avoided completely and those for which a dosage reduction is permissible. The BNF lists contraindications to treatments within each drug category, and the NPF has the same format. 'Cautions' are given, which need to be taken into account before prescribing particular drugs. The clinical relevance of such 'cautions' in individuals will often need to be discussed with a doctor.

Side-effects

Common side-effects are given within each product monograph in the BNF, but, for more detail, including those side-effects which occur rarely, the *Summary of Product Characteristics*, formerly the *Data Sheet Compendium*, can be consulted. This is available from the Association of the British Pharmaceutical Industry, but a copy should be available in every general practice. Prescribers should be familiar with common side-effects as patients will be interested in potential problems with therapy. It is often better to prepare patients for possible side-effects rather than to deal with their worried questions after they have read the patient information leaflet. Such leaflets are provided with many prescribed medicines and must be available for all medicines by 1999.

Drug interactions

Major interactions of clinical significance are given in some sections of the NPF, for example for aspirin, but not usually in the BNF. In this publication, Appendix 1 must be consulted.

Over-the-counter medicines and herbal products may interact with prescribed medicines. Prescribers should always question patients about the use of such products before prescribing. Additional information on such interactions can be obtained from pharmacists and drug information centres.

Reporting adverse drug reactions

All prescribers have an extremely important role to play in the reporting of adverse drug reactions. In the UK, a very successful scheme, known as 'the yellow card scheme', is operated jointly by the Committee on Safety of Medicines (CSM) and the Medicines Control Agency. Information is provided by the prescriber on a yellow card, which is then submitted to the scheme. Copies of yellow cards can be found at the rear of the BNF, in MIMS and in the *Summary of Product Characteristics*. They can also be obtained by dialling 100 and asking for Freephone CSM or dialling 0800 731 6789 (see 'Adverse Reactions to Drugs' in BNF).

The function of the scheme incorporates the following objectives:

- to collect reports on any reactions to a new drug
- to gather serious reactions to established products even when the cause is not definitely established

- to maintain patient and professional confidence in prescribed drugs
- to provide early warnings of previously unsuspected adverse drug reactions
- to collate and compare adverse drug reactions between medicines within the same therapeutic class
- to look for factors that predispose to adverse reactions to specific drugs.

The reporting of adverse reactions is currently limited to doctors, dentists, hospital pharmacists, Her Majesty's coroners and pilot schemes involving community pharmacists. Nurse prescribers who identify, or are suspicious, that a patient has suffered an adverse reaction to a medicinal product should ask a doctor to complete a form and check details with them before submitting it to the CSM.

It is hoped that, in the future, nurse prescribers will be able to complete these forms in their own right without requiring a doctor's signature. It is thought that only about 10 per cent of serious and fatal reactions are ever reported, and the involvement of additional health professionals could help to increase the level of reporting.

Quantities to prescribe

Quantities issued on prescription must be calculated in relation to expected 'normal' usage levels and the frequency with which the patient is seen.

Creams and ointments are often needed as emollients and soap substitutes for eczema and psoriasis sufferers. A common complaint about prescribers is that inadequate quantities of skin products are often prescribed. This results in poor compliance with therapy, flare-ups of skin conditions and probable increases in steroid usage. This is an example of short-sighted prescribing causing future and long-term problems.

Examples of realistic quantities of aqueous cream emollient for 1 month for an adult are:

- localized eczema on the arms only: 500 g
- generalized eczema over most of the body: 6 x 500 g.

As a soap substitute, additional amounts of emulsifying ointment of 500 – 1000 g will be needed, taking into account the number of washing facilities around the house, work and so on.

When prescribing wound management products, normal usage should be considered, and, for those products that can be changed once a week, a smaller number of products than has traditionally been the case should be prescribed. For example, five hydrocolloid dressings should be adequate for one month unless the patient has multiple areas of treatment or the product is being changed too frequently, when alternative products may be more suitable. In the nurse prescribing pilot scheme, the practice with the greatest cost reduction for prescribing had reviewed and rationalised the prescribing of such products within a nursing home (*Drug and Therapeutics Bulletin* Seminar 1996). The cost–benefit study (DoH 1992), prior to the pilot nurse prescribing scheme, demonstrated that nurses used dressings and other items in a cost-effective manner. It is important that regular independent educational updates are available to maintain the knowledge base necessary to support this prescribing.

Similar considerations are important for catheter and stoma care products, which comprise a huge proportion of the country's prescribing budget, with a huge potential for waste if excessive prescribing occurs. Products have expiry dates, and prefilled catheters have shorter than average dates. Stockpiling must therefore be discouraged and quantities should be based on average usage, as detailed in the *Drug Tariff*. The following examples should raise awareness of issues to consider when asked to prescribe an item in this category:

1. Re-usable Nelaton catheters for intermittent catheterisation come in packs of five. One catheter can be used for 5–7 days. One pack of five is therefore adequate for patients receiving monthly prescriptions.
2. Drainable leg bags are available in packs of 10, which is more than enough for a monthly prescription, as these have a similar life to the reusable catheters. Packs may be split if necessary.

Product selection, communication and patient compliance

Product selection

In addition to the many clinical issues involved in product selection, the prescriber must also consider ease of use and patient acceptability, which will often relate to a patient's lifestyle. However, these considerations play only a small part in achieving success with long-term therapy.

Collection of the prescription – why is this not 100 per cent?

A significant number of patients who are given a prescription in the UK never actually get it dispensed. The rate of this 'non-presentation' for GP-generated prescriptions is about 5 per cent but may be up to 20 per cent or more in elderly patients (Beardon et al. 1993). Since elderly people do not pay prescription charges, motivation rather than finance is the contributing factor. The figure relating to nurse-generated prescriptions is as yet unknown, but the comparison would be interesting. Prescribers must always remember that patients do not always feel that a prescription is appropriate for their needs.

Reasons are many and varied, but lack of satisfaction with the consultation, including inadequate explanation by the prescriber, plays a part. Good prescriber–patient communication is thus a vital part of the prescribing process.

Provision of patient information

The information given to the patient must contain sufficient detail to encourage patients not only to obtain the product prescribed, but then also to comply with therapy. The essential components of such a discussion should include the following:

- the reason for the prescription
- the name and purpose of the medicine, including whether it will treat the condition, for example paracetamol for fever

control, or just control symptoms, as do emollients in the management of eczema
- the length of treatment that will be needed before an effect is seen
- the likely total length of treatment that will be necessary
- the significance of missed doses, and necessary action
- how to recognise adverse effects
- the concurrent use of over-the-counter medicines.

Basic information on the use of the product should never be overlooked even if patients have received the product before. A good example is a patient on inhaler therapy, who may be found to have poor inhaler technique even though repeat prescriptions have been received for years.

Information on the use of nurse-prescribed items, together with GP-generated items, is also important. For example, the parent of a child with eczema may be unclear about the roles of the emollient prescribed by the nurse and the steroid cream provided by the GP or dermatologist and whether both can be applied together. These issues are often where 'seamless care', even between professionals within the same team, may falter, with resulting confusion.

Labelling of medicines

The label on the medicine must now always be computer generated by pharmacists and will contain the following information:

- the name of the product, which will be generic for nurse prescriptions, except for the few exceptions highlighted in the NPF
- the name of the patient
- the date of dispensing
- the total quantity dispensed
- the directions for use
- the name and address of the supplying pharmacy
- advice to keep the medicine out of the reach of children.

Additional information that will be added by the pharmacist, for example 'take with or after food', 'dissolve in water' and so on, is indicated in the product monograph in the NPF.

Patients may ask for further explanation of these instructions and may quickly forget the additional verbal information provided by the pharmacist at the time of issue. They may then ask the next health professional with whom they have contact. As described earlier, nurse prescribers can obtain additional information on drug therapy from many sources, but the local community pharmacist should be a valuable resource. The pharmacist can also provide more user-friendly packs, when required, to help with specific problems, for example difficulty opening standard bottles.

For patients who are identified as poor compliers, the use of individual dosing systems (such as Nomad or Manrex) could be considered. However, if poor memory is the cause of poor compliance, these methods cannot guarantee success, although they may help to guide patients who are confused by the number of medications prescribed.

Oral syringes are routinely dispensed for the administration of liquid doses for volumes less than 5 ml. (This is of particular relevance to nurse prescribers when prescribing paracetamol for post-immunisation pyrexia.)

Repeat prescribing systems and the nurse prescribing process

All efficient general practices should operate an effective repeat prescribing policy. The aim of this should be to ensure that the ordering and provision of repeat prescriptions is safe and accurate, that there is an agreed 'normal' quantity issued (28 days, 30 days, and so on.) and that patients are reviewed at an agreed frequency. This review should involve a consultation to establish the effectiveness of the medication, to monitor patients for side-effects and to confirm that there is a continuing need for the medication. All practice staff should work towards the safe operation of the system and should ensure that review dates are complied with and not over-ridden during busy times. If the review system is allowed to break down, patients rapidly fall into the habit of demanding repeats without ever seeing the original prescriber, and products are continued *ad infinitum*, with potentially disastrous results. It is stated in the *Nurse Prescribing Guidance* (NHS Executive HQ 1997) that 'the nurse should be mindful of any prescribing protocols agreed within the GP practice relevant to the patient' (p. 15). Practice protocols may need to identify items that are in the NPF but which nurses would not generally want to repeat without further consultation, for example clotrimazole cream.

The general guidance for repeat prescriptions (NHS Executive HQ 1997) is 'that no more than six repeat prescriptions should be made, or six months should elapse, whichever is the less, without re-assessing the patient's needs' (p. 14). The repeat system relies on the accurate entry of the initial prescription into the patient's medical records (often paper *and* computerised). Other prescribers in the practice may be asked to authorise future repeat prescriptions of items originally nurse prescribed. This is satisfactory provided that the original prescriber has indicated a review or reauthorisation date. The latter may be acceptable periodically for some patients and some products for which a regular chronic prescription is obtained, for example the emollients mentioned above for eczema. Such patients should still be reviewed to monitor them for infected eczema, to check progress of the eczema with the therapy provided and to give reassurance and answer the patient's questions. At two of the demonstration pilot sites for nurse prescribing, nurses conducted a review of repeat prescriptions, highlighting patients who were receiving repeat items that were in the NPF but that had originally been prescribed by doctors. At one of the sites, many products were found to be no longer required, and considerable savings were realised (Luker and Austin 1997).

Lost prescriptions or requests for duplicate prescriptions

Requests for immediate repeat prescriptions or within a few hours or days of the original issue do occur, and a strict policy should be adopted. If, after questioning the patient, the request appears to be genuine ('The bottle broke!'), a further prescription could be given and the records clearly marked.

Disposal of unwanted medicines

All prescribers should encourage the safe disposal of unwanted medicines, whether discontinued and no longer needed, or having expired. Patients should be encouraged to return such items to community pharmacists. Most participate in an official scheme using safe 'dumping' containers that are collected from the pharmacy on a regular basis and incinerated. No medication, however small in size or volume, should be disposed of in domestic or commercial refuse, and disposal via the sewerage system is illegal, even for individuals, with obvious potential dangers.

References

Barber, N. (1995) What constitutes good prescribing? *British Medical Journal* **310**: 923–5.

Beardon, P.H.G, McGilchrist, M.M., McKendrick, A.D., McDevitt, D.G. and MacDonald, T.M. (1993) *British Medical Journal* **307**: 846–8.

DoH (1992) *Nurse Prescribing – a Cost Benefit Study*. DoH, London.

Drug and Therapeutics Bulletin Seminar (1996) Nurse prescribing issues. *Pharmaceutical Journal* **257**: 764–5.

Luker, K. and Austin, L. (1997) Nurse prescribing; study findings and GP views. *Prescriber* **8**: 31–4.

NHS Executive HQ (1997) *Nurse Prescribing Guidance*, April. NHS Executive, Leeds.

5 The management of prescribing

Mark Campbell

This chapter describes some key aspects of the current framework within which primary care prescribing is both undertaken and managed, and places nurses' prescribing in context within this. A complex web of factors influences prescribing; there is therefore a wide range of management strategies. Some are determined nationally (for example, by the DoH or reflecting wider government policy), while others are locally driven at regional or health authority level. This chapter considers mainly medicines prescribed in primary care rather than treatment in hospitals or self-treatment. The terms 'drug' and 'medicine' will be used interchangeably throughout the text.

Background

Although many medicines are prescribed for symptom control in acute, self-limiting illnesses, the majority of use is probably for the treatment of common chronic diseases, for most of which drug treatment is a central feature. Prescribing therefore has a public health function – to lessen morbidity and (hopefully) reduce mortality. The pharmaceutical armamentarium increases by about 15 new drugs each year, while new clinical evidence continues to appear for existing drugs, making the choice of treatment increasingly difficult. Within this process, the NHS commits huge amounts of health care professional and patient time to prescribing. The cost of prescribing is also substantial; the GP drugs bill was, in 1997, about £4.3 billion in England, accounting for about 14 per cent of total NHS expenditure and by far the largest proportion of NHS costs after staff. This amount represents about £80 per head of population per year. For the past decade, primary care prescribing costs have risen by between 8 per cent and 14 per cent per annum, usually by at least three times the rate of increase in funding for the NHS as a whole. Promoting appropriate and effective prescribing while containing the rise in prescribing costs is therefore a considerable challenge.

Life cycle of prescription

After a prescription form (FP10 in England, GP10 in Scotland) is issued, it is dispensed either by a pharmacist, dispensing doctor or appliance contractor. The form is then sent to the Prescription Pricing Authority (PPA) for pricing and reimbursement of the drug costs and overheads to the dispensing contractor. The prescription data are also incorporated into a variety of electronic and hard copy prescribing information systems for feedback to prescribers (see below).

Drug pricing

Manufacturers' list prices for drugs (that is, those shown in the BNF or MIMS) are set by means of a joint agreement between the DoH and individual pharmaceutical companies – the Pharmaceutical Price Regulation Scheme (PPRS). Within the framework of this scheme, a price is agreed for a new drug that represents between 17 and 25 per cent profit-on-return (POR). For existing medicines, companies must apply to the DoH to increase the price of a drug. If this is agreed, the POR must nevertheless remain within the target range. Increases in the price of existing drugs are unusual; at present, there is no, or a slightly negative, drug price inflation. Arguably, the PPRS maintains the price of drugs at artificially high levels, but such arguments neglect the importance of the domestic pharmaceutical industry to the UK economy. For example, the pharmaceutical industry is the UK's second largest exporter by worth (in excess of £2 billion per annum) and a large provider of high-calibre employment. However, one consequence of the PPRS is that drugs with essentially similar therapeutic effects may vary considerably in price. For example, the world's biggest-selling pharmaceutical, the anti-ulcer drug ranitidine (Zantac, Glaxo), has only minor pharmacological and clinical differences compared with cimetidine (Tagamet, SmithKline Beecham) yet costs over 20 per cent more.

In the UK, hospitals may buy some drugs at considerable discount; such discounts are not available in primary care, but, unlike for hospitals, VAT is not charged on drugs. Since the choice of drug in hospitals often influences prescribing in primary care, there is a potential problem when the drug of choice is determined by that which can be bought at highest discount but may have the highest list price, which is then borne by GPs who have to continue treatment.

Prescription charges

Although controversial, most countries with state-funded health care systems have some form of prescription tax or 'co-payment'. In the UK, this is a flat-rate levy, unrelated to the cost of the individual prescription drug. In some other countries, patients pay a proportion of the cost of the drug, usually up to a maximum payment. Increases in prescription charges are thought to have an impact on the number of prescriptions dispensed (but not necessarily the number issued), and there is concern that charges act as disincentive to have prescriptions dispensed. Nevertheless, prescription charges remain a significant source of revenue (about £300 million annually). There is a long-running debate over exemption from charges on the grounds of chronic illness, age or income (or whether there should be charges at all), and the current framework contains many inconsistencies. However, a better system has yet to emerge.

Selected list

Some countries operate mandatory or voluntary national formularies of 'preferred' drugs. In the UK, this policy has never gained much favour; instead, some drugs, usually on the basis of limited clinical value, are prohibited from FP10 prescription and other drugs in the same class promoted as alternatives. In 1985, the first selected list (then called a limited list) was published, in which some benzodiazepines, cough medicines and vitamin preparations became non-prescribable at NHS expense. The policy probably achieved some economies but was very unpopular among GP prescribers and patients. It has only operated in one therapeutic area since – topical non-steroidal anti-inflammatory drugs – where it has been implemented slightly differently. A maximum treatment cost (or reference price) was set, based upon the lowest-price preparation available. Any preparation that cost more than this maximum would not be prescribable; all manufacturers subsequently adjusted the price of their products downwards to this level.

Financial incentives

Prior to 1991, there was no upper (or lower) limit on GP prescribing costs. However, the 1991 NHS White Paper introduced indicative prescribing amounts (IPAs), which were the best estimate of a practice's prescribing needs for a year. For practices that elected to be fundholders, the IPA became a real cash amount, and savings on the practice fund, of which the IPA was one element, could be retained and reinvested in improving local patient services. Subsequently, in 1993, this incentive was extended to non-fundholders. The impact of these schemes has been evaluated, and, although the picture is not clear cut, some important principles have emerged:

- Financial incentives are effective in improving budgetary discipline; fundholders have consistently out-performed non-fundholders at budget adherence, although whether this is because they have received a disproportionately large budget share is unclear.
- Fundholder and non-fundholder savings were generally made by simple means, such as increased generic prescribing.
- The reductions in cost growth achieved by fundholders were not, overall, sustainable, and, in studies, cost growth among fundholders and non-fundholders was eventually similar.

Financial incentives are now an integral part of practice prescribing allocations; more recently, incentive schemes for non-fundholders have included additional, local, prescribing quality criteria that practices have had to satisfy before the incentive payments can be made. One constant criticism of financial incentives is that they depend on the method used to determine the practice prescribing allocation. Originally, historical patterns of expenditure were used to determine these, but, more recently, most practice allocations have been set with reference to a local capitation benchmark. Practices with high baseline per capita costs receive a lower than average increase in allocation year-on-year, and vice versa. Although imperfect, this system is an improvement on the earlier methods. Most health authorities also incorporate a degree of sophistication in taking account of local practice circumstances such as high-cost specialist drug costs and residential and nursing home patients. From April 1999, there will be a major change to the financial framework for primary care prescribing, with the introduction of primary care groups that will cover, on average, a population of 100,000. Prescribing allocations, which will be cash limited, will instead be made at the level of the primary care group, which will also be responsible for any overspend.

Prescribing information and feedback

Prior to 1988, there was little feedback to individual GPs on their own prescribing habits and no detailed information for the monitoring of prescribing at any level other than regional or national. The introduction of prescription analysis and cost (PACT) reports, which followed the computerisation of the PPA, has allowed an increased awareness both of variations in prescribing and of trends. PACT has become a generic description of prescription information at different levels of organisational detail (GPs, practices, health authority, regional and national) and drug detail (preparations, drugs, therapeutic areas and total prescribing) and available in different media to different users. GPs receive a hard copy summary each quarter, whereas health authorities and other NHS organisations now have electronic access at a level of detail appropriate to their needs.

The impact of PACT is impossible to determine. At the very least, it has played a part in raising awareness of prescribing issues, in particular the variation between practices and areas, in some cases prompting further investigation of underlying variations in morbidity. Although comprehensive, timely and understandable, PACT reports do not yet provide sufficient detail to understand fully the complexity of prescribing. In particular, the system is focused upon the drug prescribed; patient data (for example, age, sex and diagnosis) are not yet being collected. In order to overcome this, PACT data have been used to derive simple prescribing indicators that might, for example, be based on the choice of drugs in a therapeutic group or the level of prescribing of drugs where there is only limited evidence of efficacy.

A further problem that indirectly affects PACT is the increasing trend of buying medicines over the counter in pharmacies and of private prescriptions. Since these items are not routinely captured, PACT is incomplete as a global record of medicine utilisation.

Evidence-based medicine, guidelines, protocols and formularies

The evaluation of available evidence in order to support prescribing decision-making is both difficult and very time consuming. One of the most common ways of implementing evidence-based decisions is by means of written guidelines, protocols or drug formularies, in which treatments are recommended only if supported by good research evidence.

Such initiatives are usually local, at the level of a health authority, or sometimes within an individual GP practice. Hospitals have traditionally had local drug formularies; more recently, some GP practices have devised their own formularies. Although in theory an attractive way of making objective guidance available to a large audience, guidelines and protocols often fail to be successfully introduced and used.

Common problems include: their not being seen as locally relevant; end-users not feeling that they have 'ownership' of the guidelines; and the guidelines being cumbersome in use, for example an encyclopaedia-sized publication when a pocket-sized guide is needed. A particular problem arises when, as in some areas of nursing care, only limited or poor-quality research evidence is available. In such cases, guidelines based on the consensus opinion of 'national' experts may be received poorly by individual practitioners, each of whom perceives him- or herself also to have at least as much expertise and/or experience.

Face-to-face contact

The various management strategies are mainly implemented through health authorities and their professional prescribing advisers (doctors and pharmacists). These advisers are responsible for setting and monitoring prescribing allocations as well as promoting high-quality, cost-effective prescribing. Face-to-face contact is known to be the most effective behaviour change strategy, but the opportunity for this, with the average health authority having two advisers and up to 100 or more practices, is limited. Increasingly, other professionals, such as community pharmacists and specialist nurses, are being used to assist practices in changing their prescribing practice.

Repeat prescribing

Since most medicines are used for chronic disease, they are given long term. This means that a high proportion of drugs are given as repeat prescriptions, so the organisation of practice systems for their issue is a potential source of improving long-term drug treatment and reducing inappropriate usage. Repeat prescriptions are usually defined as those for drugs that have already been initiated and subsequently repeated without a face-to-face consultation with a doctor. Although many patients on (often multiple) repeat prescriptions are not adequately reviewed, there is no universally agreed 'model' system for achieving this. Most initiatives to improve repeat prescribing have been locally driven and, because of the size of the task, usually concentrate on a specific therapeutic area, for example ulcer-healing drugs.

Compliance and waste

Estimates of the rate of primary non-compliance (prescriptions being issued but not dispensed) are between 5–20 per cent. Even worse, when prescriptions have been dispensed, only a half are taken as intended. The reasons for this are complex and outside the scope of this chapter, but non-compliance is a major concern for which the solutions are preventing inappropriate prescribing and providing better information for patients through counselling by health care professionals. Non-compliance also leads to waste; local DUMP (Disposal of Unwanted Medicines) campaigns frequently collect tons of unwanted and unused drugs. District nurses and health visitors are in a unique position to detect the 'hoarding' of medicines by house-bound patients and, at present, are probably underused in helping to address this problem.

Postgraduate education and training

There is a wide range of provision of postgraduate education, including that on therapeutics, for GPs in the UK, some of it arranged formally through regional postgraduate deans who are responsible for accrediting appropriate educational events under the Post Graduate Education Allowance scheme. This is a financial incentive for GPs to accrue a specified amount of approved educational time each year. However, the vast majority of the postgraduate education and training events on therapeutics is sponsored by, and may be delivered by, the pharmaceutical industry. There is an obvious conflict of interest in such events, although, in many cases, they are organised on a non-promotional basis. There is a need to ensure that nurse prescribers have adequate access to appropriate training on prescribing and therapeutics issues, which may be covered in only a rudimentary fashion in the basic training course.

Generic prescribing

Generic (non-brand) forms of a drug are produced once the patent life of a branded medicine has expired. They are of similar quality and often cost considerably less. Their use is one feature of good prescribing. The increase in generic prescribing rates during the past 10 years has been one of the few 'sea changes' in prescribing. About 60 per cent of prescriptions are currently written generically compared with only 40 per cent in 1991, and the rate in some health authorities and for some individual drugs is substantially higher. The financial savings arising from this over the past 7 years are difficult to estimate, but nationally the amount is probably measured in tens of millions of pounds. For a very small number of drugs, including some modified-release preparations, generic prescribing is not appropriate. It may also be a problem for some products prescribed by nurses, for example appliances and dressings.

The pharmaceutical industry

Overall, the pharmaceutical industry represents a very successful and profitable business. Its research and development activities have produced drugs that have reduced morbidity and mortality. It is also very skilful at promoting its products. It would seem prudent therefore to exercise a degree of caution in relationships between the NHS and the pharmaceutical industry. For example, claims made for new drugs or preparations often require further scrutiny; at the time of launch, the available evidence may, for example, be incomplete. All NHS staff, including nurses, have a duty to maintain high standards of professional business conduct. There is, understandably, considerable sensitivity, both within the DoH, and at various levels of the NHS, to the possibility of improper influences on prescribing.

Nurse prescribing

As well as being a significant personal and professional development for nurses, nurse prescribing is also another strategy for improving prescribing. It ought to save time (and therefore cost), reduce waste and possibly lead to a better management of conditions for which GPs' skills and experience are perceived to be limited but where nurses are usually heavily involved in care, such as wound management, incontinence and stoma care. Interim results of the evaluation of the pilot nurse prescribing sites are encouraging, although the range of drugs in the NPF is as yet probably too small (particularly for practice nurses) for significant changes to be detected.

6 Keep taking your medication or you will not get better. Who is the non-compliant patient?

Joel Richman

The concept of the non-compliant patient is a product of what Foucault (1976) calls the 'medical gaze', a clinical construct embedded in its practical and ideological perspective which states that patients who do not follow doctors' orders must be deviants. Non-compliance covers a range of assumed patient behaviour: those who misuse prescribed medication, fail to change their lifestyles to alleviate illness, or neglect clinical attendance. We shall examine the medication aspect here, primarily based on research relating to doctors' consultations. It has obvious reference and significance for prescribing nurses, who must not automatically assume that all their patients will be happy to follow their instructions, because nurses might adhere more to a 'social model' of medicine.

The chapter will attempt to locate the social conditions conducive for non-compliance; this includes styles of consultation in general and psychiatric medicine. The next purpose is to outline the strategies used to produce patient conformity and to raise some of the ethical implications of these. Finally, the patient's view is posited, elaborating the complexities of lay reasoning about illness, in which its existential qualities linking to medication are mapped out. Illness is intimately wrapped round notions of the self, disturbing its favourable presentation. Medication is a symbolic and practical intrusion, often adding another conflicting dimension to the self's attempts not to be defined by illness *per se*.

A non-compliant patient becomes deviant because he or she has violated one of the cardinal principles of the Parsonian (1951) sick role. The patient is obliged not only to seek out medical assistance when ill, but also passively to accept doctors' instructions regarding the managing of the illness, especially concerning medication regimes. Another patient duty is not to linger in the sick role beyond the doctor's legitimate expectations. This deviance also includes 'overcompliance' – the taking of unnecessary medication. Those who are unemployed find comfort and respectable status in the sick role. Those who cannot accept that their condition is a result of normal ageing also 'overmedicate'. Combined with the ideology of the sick role is the Weberian prostestant ethic (Weber 1947): we live in an economic, cost-effective world. The non-compliant patient has also violated the expertise and labours of the medical practitioner. That is why 'overdosers' on prescribed medication in accident and emergency departments are often referred to as 'rubbish' cases, unnecessarily wasting the time of clinical staff who could be deployed better. Some (for example, Britten 1994) prefer the term 'adherence' rather than 'compliance', indicating more the patients' choice in issues of medication. Here, we stick with compliance, the term more generally used, bearing in mind its ideological bias and that conformists and non-conformists do not constitute two polarised positions: a patient can be compliant with one medical regime but not another.

Consultation styles

Szasz and Hollender (1956) were among the first to recognise that the Parsonian ideal-type model of the doctor–patient relationship was not the only one. Each style had implications for patient compliance.

The *authoritarian* consultation projects the image that patients are clinically 'insignificant'; if patients do not accept the style, they should get another doctor, and patients talk when 'requested'. The doctor gives only that information which he or she thinks is relevant, and patients are not encouraged to question clinical data. The inherent antagonistic relationship resulting is not conducive to compliance.

The *permissive* style (verging on *laissez-faire*) also does not generate patient compliance. Doctors are always seeking to please the patient, leading to unstructured sessions that make it difficult for the patient to get comprehensive information and that submerge the treatment goal.

The *psychotherapeutic* style assumes that patients' fears about treatment and medication are not genuine everyday ones. Instead, clients' responses are interpreted in a therapeutic way. Patients' questions resisting prescribed medication are interpreted as the product of unconscious motives, for example as a resistance to a father figure. There is a valuable lesson for nurses about the above style: do not indulge in 'therapy talk' to confuse medication requirements.

The *participatory* style (Korsch 1969) produces high rates of compliance (as it does in experimental group dynamics). Here, doctors assume that patients have rights to question and complain. The medical regime is tailored to the patient's everyday routine; in a way that is realistic. This style is sometimes welded on to doctor–patient contracts, emphasising mutual responsibilities. Patients are best able to evaluate the doctor's human relations skills rather than technical ones. Bond and Salinger (1979) have shown that joint prescribing with psychiatrist and pharmacist for those with schizophrenia produces a higher rate of compliance. Patients' complaints are not treated as delusions or signs of denial but as real problems. Drug dosages are rapidly modified to cause fewer side-effects, especially tardive dyskinesia and Parkinsonian effects. Poor control of the side-effects of psychotropic drugs is a major reason for non-compliance.

Evidence of non-compliance

There is no simple and uniform way of measuring non-compliance. Counting the pills left in a container and measuring the medicine level in a bottle both suffer from obvious defects. Stichele (1991, p. 30) argues that:

> Pill count grossly overestimates compliance, and misses some 10 per cent of overt non-compliers. False positive assessment of compliance occurs when patients deliberately discard tablets, before returning containers. This is called 'pill dumping' or the 'parking lot' phenomenon.

The measurement of metabolite level is also not always a predictor: for example, those with bipolar affective disorder (manic depression) are stabilised on lithium carbonate, but the latter's absorption rate is extremely high. Drug testing in prisons has similar problems: heroin leaves little trace after 30 hours; marijuana, in contrast, is detectable up to 30 days after first taking it. Patient interviews are also notoriously unreliable. A founding father of ancient Greek medicine, Hippocrates, warned of patients' lies over 2,500 years ago. Mothers will lie on behalf of sick children lest they are not considered 'good mothers'. Sheiner *et al.* (1974) have demonstrated that doctors very frequently overestimate the compliance levels of their own patients as a psychological boost to their own prestige. There are lessons here for the new, prescribing nurses, wanting medical acclaim for their skills.

A recent method for evaluating compliance is the addition to the prescribed medication of another low-dose substance as a pharmacological marker, one which is easily detected in blood or urine samples. Low dosages of digoxin were used in Finnish heart studies as part of the Karelia public health programme in the 1980s. In most Western developed nations, patients must consent to the use of pharmacological markers because, strictly speaking, they are not integral to the medication regime. Other pharmacological markers have been suggested: radioactive substances; inert molecules, for example perfluorocarbon; stable isotopes, for example C-glucose or C-benzoid acid; and low-dose phenobarbitone of 2mg/day, used because of its half-life of 4 days in adults. Patients are generally more conformist when they are informed that they are going to have, for example, a blood or urine test as part of their care plan. Without pharmacological markers, blood levels *per se* are very inaccurate: the latter is affected by body mass:fat ratios, gastric acidity levels and so on. A new generation of electronic monitoring devices is coming on the market, for example aerosol sprays that activate external, graduated scales (very much on the same principle as longlife batteries, allowing the user to know how much power is left). In addition to the extra expense, it is still not possible to say that the user has used the spray effectively for his or her particular condition. When counselling is built into treatment regimes, patients become more 'honest' about their compliance rates, as indicated in hypertension studies in the USA.

Some features of non-compliance

Studies of non-compliance indicate the following:

- Anyone can be a non-compliant patient. Doctors themselves are notorious for being non-compliant when ill.
- The number of articles on non-compliance has been doubling every 5 years, indicating how seriously the medical profession regards the theme.
- The proportion of patients who fail to comply fully with prescribed treatment is around 30–60 per cent. With some medicines, this can be as high as 90 per cent.
- When patients fail to improve on medication, doctors tend to resort to blaming the patient (victim) for not taking the medication correctly. Carmeli's (1976) study of doctor–patient relationships in a diabetic clinic demonstrated that doctors' diagnostic reasoning was akin to that of magic used in tribal society. It was a ritualised, closed system of thought excluding the scientific possibility that, for example, the batch of insulin used by patients was faulty. Instead, the patient was regarded as the cause of the 'malevolence' regarding the fluctuation of glucose level displayed. The newly introduced human insulin was automatically assumed by the medical establishment to be better than the long-used insulin derived from pigs. Again, patients' complaints about it were dismissed as 'not possible' for the new insulin matched better the human condition. Later research showed that patients' doubts were correct: the human insulin gave less body warning about sinking into hypoglycaemic attacks.
- Non-compliance is far more than misunderstanding (bad communication) between doctor and patient, although Ley *et al.* (1976) have shown that, on leaving clinics and surgeries, patients forget 37–54 per cent of information that they have been given.
- Non-compliance is not related solely to social class, marital status, age or IQ: even children can cheat. Belmonte (1981) showed how diabetic children cheated when taken away to summer camp. It was assumed that the children would be more conformist to the strict, diabetic, self-administered regime in groups, which would establish conformist norms of behaviour.

Instead, children falsified their sugar level readings, believing, logically, that if their level were 'low', they were recovering. Many adults also have a 'make-believe' attitude to their own illness, 'willing it to their order'.

- Non-compliance is more likely to be a 'problem' (a) if drugs are taken over a long period of time, and (b) the more drugs are prescribed, with varying frequency of ingestion.

- Compliance is poor if medication is expensive. (This does not apply primarily to the UK.) This is especially true in less-developed nations: the poor, who have to pay a considerable part of their meagre income on drugs, will tend to dilute medication to make it 'last longer'. Many of the medicines for sale could also be out of date. The same behaviour occurs with poor blacks in the USA ghettos: they will frequently not take prescriptions to be dispensed. It should be noted that approximately 40 million Americans have no health insurance.

- There is a much higher level of compliance if the disease (for example some sexually transmitted diseases) is short term, symptomatic, painful and publicly distressing.

- Compliance is poor if 'side-effects' are severe. In fact, there is no such thing as a 'side-effect', only the effects of the drugs. Drugs for hypertension are known to make the patient feel worse; 40 per cent of the USA population has high blood pressure, unbeknown to them, and hypertension, if untreated, is a 'silent killer'. What can be listed as severe side-effects varies according to personal judgement. Some patients stop taking chlorpromazine for schizophrenia because they put on weight. In fact, the drug does not cause weight increase but makes patients very thirsty, many then drinking heavily sugared soft drinks. This latter effect is a latent aspect of the medication. Psychiatric nurses locked into the medical model of care very often become concerned only about the frequency of dosage, neglecting social drinking habits.

- Those at the extremes of age tend to be among the most non-compliant. Those over 65 years are the major consumers of medicine because of their increasing chronicity. However, their diminishing mental and visual competence makes it difficult for many to read, follow prescribing instructions and discriminate the colours of pills. By the year 2001, there will be one million people aged over 85 years in the UK, three-quarters of whom will be women; most of this age group will live alone. About 25 per cent will develop Alzheimer's disease and other severe dementias. Many will also be physically unable to open child-proof medication containers. Physical and cognitive impairment is not the only factor behind aged non-compliance. Many have, during their life-time, experienced the fad of new 'miracle drugs' and hence are sceptical of the hyped claims being made for recent drugs. Some, not only the aged, develop the fear of becoming 'addicted' to their medication or of its poisoning them. Donovan and Blake (1992) reported that about 20 per cent of their sample of rheumatology patients gave the fear of 'addiction' as a reason for their non-compliance. The increased media attention on addiction to medications for depression by women prescribed Atavan has created moral panics wider than the drug focused upon. There is also a parallel with the scare stories about oral contraceptives, although the medical risks associated with these are very small.

- Compliance is very high in situations where people have life-threatening diseases and are offered experimental treatment as the only hope. Fox (1959) described a metabolic ward where patients became 'quasi-colleagues' to their doctors. The latter gave patients maximum information as they wanted them to be reliable monitors of the effects of the new drug. Doctors very often named their patients in resulting publications, thanking them for enduring so much discomfort for the sake of the experiments.

- Patient's knowledge of disease and treatment is not always conducive to medication conformity. Dialysis patients are very knowledgeable but are often non-compliant, especially immediately before commencing dialysis treatment on machines and as teenagers. The one aspect they most conform to is that of the phosphate-binding medicine (for preventing heart attacks). There is little association between supportive family networks and compliance (yet network support was often a criterion for 'rationing' dialysis when the technique was in its infancy). The supportive network will support the patient no matter what the dialysand does. However, the degree to which the patient regards his or her behaviour as being disruptive of family life in general is more related to compliance (Cummings 1982).

Ethnicity and compliance

As yet, very little research has been done illustrating compliance in different ethnic groups. One of the relevant issues is that many from multicultural backgrounds have lay beliefs of health different from the assumptions of the Western bioscientific model. For example, many Afro-Caribbeans have an *externalising* health belief system (Table 6.1). That is, their notion of medical causation lies outside the body, often being of a personalistic nature. This, as Richman (1987, p. 12) says:

> explains disease etiology by the 'purposeful' interventions of agents deliberately pursuing their victims, causing them to fall ill. The malevo- lence can be human [witches], non-human [ancestors and other spirits] or 'supernatural' [deities].

The belief is that, by breaking some values of moral order, the external causation of illness will then target them. They also believe that others can target misfortune on them. The body in an externalising belief system is therefore a receptacle for the illness. In Western society, the body is mainly the source of illness pathology. The bioscientific model has an *internalising* health belief system (Table 6.1), often 'fighting' illness by developing a new chemical drug level producing a body equilibrium. It is relevant to point out that most UK natives also have an external- ising lay belief model of illness causation. I have frequently heard from people with depression that the source of their complaint is partly retribution, and that depression, like a huge mist, wrapped itself around them so that they became lost.

Thus, in a internalising psychiatric setting, an Afro-Caribbean will get irritated by the psychiatrist's 'Sherlock Holmes' style of diagnosis. Give her the clues (symptoms) and she will make the diagnosis. Afro-Caribbeans have another purpose. They know the causation of their illness, very often attributed to Obeah, a 'malev- olent spirit', who has poisoned them, but they want the psychia- trist to tell them *who* has been responsible for directing Obeah towards them. The great limitation of the bioscientific model is that it is not in business to answer the questions frequently asked by all patients, for example 'Why has cancer attacked me'. The 'Why me?' stance questions one of the reasons for the

Table 6.1 Health beliefs

	Internalising	Externalising
1. Source of illness	Within the body, for example a virus	Outside the body, for example tension in relationships breaking moral codes
2. Causation	Multiple	Fewer, for example the same cause having multiple disease effects
3. Proof of improvement	Empirical scientific	Symbolic
4. Body	Complex physical	Simple; for example the body differentiation is often a 'black box' and a receptacle for disease
5. Practitioner	Treats the individual client; passivity expected	Treats the individual as part of sets of relationships to reconcile disharmony
6. Health knowledge	Monopoly of specialists	Widely dispersed in society, which gives clients great 'pull' on healers
7. Society	Complex division of labour, producing economic surpluses that support the élites	Simple division of labour, little surplus, very small 'leisured' élite or literati
8. Recovery from illness	When fit for work	When restored to the moral order of the group group. For example the Cheyenne have a 7-day singing ceremony for the ill, each verse historically recreating the universe; then the sick person is finally incorporated into it

'overdiagnosis' of Afro-Caribbeans (especially male) with schizo-phrenia. When they talk of poisoning in the consultation, this is immediately latched on to by the psychiatrist as a symptom of the illness – penetration of the body boundary is a Rank Schneider symptom of schizophrenia. Thus those with externalising health beliefs cannot conceptualise that Western, prescribed medication can cure them. They want the doctor to defend them against the outside evil force; they cannot conceptualise how a small pill will do that.

Strategies for compliance

Many strategies have been devised to overcome non-compliance:

- The use of fixed ratio combinations of medication, especially pills, simplifying the usual counting of mixed quantities of pills.
- Patient Package Inserts (PPIs) of 'full' information by the phar-maceutical company, including details of clinical trials and adverse effects ratios, slotted into the packaging. Again, it was assumed that better informed patients are compliant. Pressure from the American Medical Association had PPIs discontinued on the grounds that they were 'disrupting doctor–patient relations', that is, patients became more questioning of doctors' prescribing.
- Written contracts with patients setting out joint responsibilities. These originated in the USA, where discontented patients more often sue their practitioners.
- Counselling. This has been a difficult variable to evaluate, because there are so many different types of counselling, provided by different sources. That carried out by prescribing nurses in a clinic or home is different from that of a specialist therapist. Colcher and Bass (1972) showed that counselling parents on the use of penicillin given to their children resulted in 20 per cent more adherence than occurred in those who were not counselled.
- Coercion, or forced medication, introduced by public pressure after some mentally ill patients killed after stopping medication. Supervised discharge (s. 23 of the Mental Health Act 1983) was introduced in April 1996. The patient's recognized medical officer has the power to place patients under supervised

discharge if it is likely that they are a substantial risk to their own and others' safety. Patients can be required to attend hospital for medication. Psychiatric nurses also have the right to 'take and convey' patients to such places. Supervision registers are held by individual Trusts at local level. The facts are that psychiatric patients discharged into the community have murdered at the rate of 18 persons, usually family members, per year; the overall murder rate is about 800 persons for annum, most being carried out by those without a mental disorder. It is obvious that compulsory medication can split a professional– patient relationship based on trust.

● Financial incentives for compliance are on the agenda. In the 1970s, Austria used them as a device for mothers' compliance with antenatal sessions; the infant mortality rate fell as a result. France, with its diminishing population, has, since 1945, used attendance payments. Giuffrida and Torgerson (1997) have reviewed the financial schemes: 'The incentives ranged from relatively small amounts of money ($5) up to gifts of nearly $1,000 for a treatment programme for cocaine dependency' (p. 705). Other schemes, all in the USA, have been for antituberculosis regimes (TB is increasing, with the rise in the number of homeless, and so on), to promote anti- hypertensive treatment, for weight-reducing programmes and for paediatric outpatient attendance. Ethical issues emerge with the use of financial incentives: how much is to come out of health budgets for them?, which conditions should be supported?, is cost-effectivesness to be the only consideration? For example, homeless people with TB can quickly spread it to the host population.

Subjects' rationale for non-compliance

Non-compliant patients can have sophisticated belief systems structuring their behaviour. Conrad's (1985) study of epileptics is an illustration of this. Patients frequently know that doctors have had difficulty in matching medication levels to their condition. Self-regulation is thus an attempt to round off the doctor's incomplete knowledge, to normalise themselves. Self-regulation mimics the doctor's prescribing fiat of 'try it and see' but is more finely tuned to individual needs. Self-regulation attempts to bring a sense of order to the body with its illness, which can appear hostile, uncontrollable and rebellious – all features undermining the self. The bioscientific model often treats illness as a thing, a reification separate from sensate experience, hence the doctor's oft-repeated gambit to the patient, 'What is it that brings you here today', as an opening greeting.

Conclusion

We have stressed that non-compliance is an ideological feature of the medical model, which has to compete with other worlds in which the patient engages – sex, leisure, work, family and so on. That is why it is impossible to produce the identity profile of the non-compliant patient. Whether the prescribing nurse will have extra time to explore patients' other worlds which link with medication remains to be seen: the average GP consultation lasts about 6 minutes. We must also not forget the overcompliant patient. Hulka *et al.* (1975) discovered that doctors were not aware of 19 per cent of medications that patients were taking. This is an issue with ethnic minorities who use, for example, both traditional healers (hakims) and the GP for the same complaint. Let Hulka close for us:

> The problem of non-compliance will remain with us, it is, after all part of the human condition. It will not be, and probably should not be, conquered together. Because many prescribed medications are not powerful over and above their placebo effects, non-compliance often does no harm. When patients refuse to do what physicians advise, as expressions of their own informed free will, it is also unclear that harm has been done.
>
> (p. 858)

References

Belmonte, T. (1981) Problem of cheating in diabetic child and adolescent. *Diabetic Care* 7: 11–19.
Bond, C.A. and Salinger, P. (1979) Fluphenazine outpatient clinics, a pharmacist's role. *Journal of Clinical Psychiatry* 22: 501–3.

Britten, N. (1994) Patients' ideas about medicines: a qualitative study in a general practice population. *British Journal of General Practitioners* **44**: 465–8.

Carmeli, T. (1976) Magical elements in orthodox medicine: diabetes as a medical thought system. Paper presented to the British Medical Sociological conference at York.

Colcher, I.S. and Bass, J.W. (1972) Penicillin treatment of streptococcal pharyngitis. A comparison of schedules and the role of specific counselling. *Journal of the American Medical Association* **222**: 657–70.

Conrad, P. (1985) The meaning of medications: another look at compliance. *Social Science and Medicine* **20**: 29–37.

Cummings, K.M. (1982) Psychosocial features affecting adherence to medical regimes in a group of hemodialysis patients. *Medical Care* **10**: 567–95.

Donovan, J.L. and Blake, D.R. (1992) Patient non-compliance: deviance or reasoned decision making? *Social Science and Medicine* **34**: 507–13.

Foucault, M. (1976) *The Birth of the Clinic*. Tavistock, London.

Fox, R. (1959) *Experiment Perilous*. Free Press, Glencoe, IL.

Giuffrida, A. and Torgerson, D.J. (1997) Should we pay the patient? Review of financial incentives to enhance patient compliance. *British Medical Journal* **315**: 703–7.

Hulka, B.S., Cassel, J.C., Gupper, L.L. and Efird, R.L. (1975) Communication, compliance and concordance between physician outpatients with prescribed medications. *American Journal of Public Health* **66**: 847–58.

Korsch, S. (1969) Gaps in doctor patient communication. *New England Journal of Medicine* **76**: 42–51.

Ley, P., Bradshaw, D.W., Kincey, J.A. and Atherton, T.S. (1976) Increasing patient satisfaction with communication. *British Journal of Social and Clinical Psychology* **15**: 403–13.

Parsons, T. (1951) *The Social System*. Free Press, Glencoe, IL.

Richman, J. (1987) *Medicine and Health*. Longman, Harlow.

Sheiner, L.B., Rosenberg, B., Marathe, V.V. and Peck, C. (1974) Differences in serum digoxin concentrations between outpatients and inpatients: an effect of compliance? *Clinical Pharmacological Therapy* **15**: 239–46.

Stichele, R.V. (1991) Measurement of patient compliance and the interpretation of randomized clinical trials. *European Journal of Clinical Pharmcology* **41**: 27–35.

Szasz, T.T. and Hollender, M.H. (1956) Contributions to the philosophy of medicine. The basic models of the doctor–patient relationship. *Archives of Internal Medicine* **97**: 585–92.

Weber, M. (1947) *The Theory of Social and Economic Organisation*. Free Press, New York.

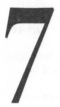

Nurse prescribing: the reality

Lorraine Berry and Rita Hurst

Dr Saul and Partners were chosen as one of the eight national pilot sites for nurse prescribing in May 1994. The commitment to the cause of nurse prescribing and the willingness to participate in data collection and evaluation at all stages were essential criteria for selection for the pilot sites (DoH 1989).

Dr Saul and Partners is a first-wave fundholding practice with a practice population of 8,500 patients. The practice consists of four GPs and two practice nurses, and is situated on a busy main road 1.5 miles north of Bolton town centre in an urban residential location. One of the practice nurses has a district nursing qualification so was able to participate in the scheme.

The housing in the practice catchment area is predominantly pre-war, comprising many terraced streets surrounded by roads of pre-war semi-detached properties; there is also a large council estate. The practice population is of mixed socio-economic class, with a 2 per cent population of ethnic minorities. The district nurses and health visitors attached to the practice are employed by Community Health Care Bolton NHS Trust and are based at a health centre that lies approximately half a mile from the surgery.

The practice has a good relationship with the Trust and the attached community staff. The GPs at the practice recognise the skills of the nurses and would agree with the statement of Carlisle (1989) that the practice of the doctor having to 'rubber stamp' a prescribing decision taken by the nurse was demeaning to both nurse and doctor; in addition, we found that this process wasted a considerable amount of time.

When the eight pilot sites were announced, we were unprepared for the amount of media attention that became focused upon us as a team. Suddenly, we were being asked to give interviews for the radio, local newspapers and nursing publications. After the initial excitement and the surge of publicity, the four participants – two district nurses, one health visitor and one practice nurse – had to prepare for the training course. It was at this stage that the reality set in and the real anxieties began to emerge.

Although we knew that the nursing profession would be closely monitoring prescribing practices, we did not initially appreciate the impact that being part of the pilot would have on us personally: it seemed the eyes of the nursing profession were following our every move.

We had a limited time to complete the open learning component before the 2-day course, and there was certainly a sense of panic when we were about to take the written examination. With the eyes of the country upon us, the fear of failure was very worrying.

On reflection, although the course seemed rushed, the content was adequate for the formulary as it stands at present. We could anticipate the potential benefits of prescribing, for both patients and professionals. Having waited 8 years for nurse prescribing to become a reality, the four of us in Bolton were determined to make it viable.

The Nurse Prescribers' Formulary

The NPF was not allocated to us until the day we actually started prescribing (3 October 1994); however, the recommendation in the Crown Report (DoH 1989) gave some insight into its content. To some community nurses, the NPF seemed very limiting and would possibly not provide enough scope to have any great impact on the delivery of patient care. However, over the 12-month pilot project, it was not just the actual content of what we were able to prescribe, nor the newly acquired prescribing status we had attained, but the enhanced approach to patient care that offered the most potential.

The NPF seemed to benefit the district nurses more than health visitors or practice nurses. The majority of the day-to-day items used by district nurses are in the formulary. Products for wound care, catheter care and bowel management, all areas that are generally managed by district nurses, are covered by the NPF. For the health visitors and practice nurses, the NPF is more limiting.

During the pilot study, we were asked to identify products that we thought should be included in the formulary, for example saline nose drops, Sudocrem, eye drops, Diprobase, Infacol, soya products and Flamazine. As a result of the evaluation study of the eight pilot sites, Luker *et al.* (1997) recommended that consideration should be given to the range of preparations for inclusion in the new NPF as it was recognised that the original NPF might be restricting practice and further evaluation was required in order to allow nurses to achieve greater autonomy and, as a result, to enhance patient care delivery.

Accountability and responsibility

When the four of us in Bolton qualified as nurse prescribers, we recognised that this new role added another facet to our accountabilities. We realised that the legal implications of nurse prescribing meant that, in a court of law, our actions would be compared against those of a reasonable doctor rather than a reasonable nurse (Tingle 1990). Hunt (1988) also concludes that, if a doctor can be sued for failing to warn about risks, equally a nurse can if he or she assumes the doctor's role. As new nurse prescribers, we felt quite anxious about the extra responsibility and accountability that signing prescriptions would place on us. Accountability not only means having to answer for an action when something goes wrong, but is also a continuous process of monitoring how we perform professionally (Tschudin 1986). We were able to overcome some of our anxieties by meeting weekly and incorporating peer group review. Pearson (1987) defined peer review as:

> A process used to appraise the quality of a nurse's professional performance and is conducted by a group of nurses who are actively engaged in some component of practice.

During the peer review sessions, while maintaining patient confidentiality, we discussed patient case studies and the issues of prescribing. These sessions offered us the opportunity to discuss each other's roles and clarify responsibilities; in turn, the working relationships and communication within the primary health care team were strengthened. It was not only the prescribing nurses, but also the staff nurses and non-prescribing practice nurse who were included in these sessions, and they also contributed their opinions and ideas on nurse prescribing. Being accountable for our prescribing decisions made us reflect more on our professional practice and our holistic approach to patient care.

Surprisingly, despite the anxieties and pressures resulting from piloting this project, prescribing very quickly became a routine part of our role and was easily absorbed into working practice. The following text will look at prescribing from a district nurse nursing perspective.

District nurse

As the district nurse attached to Dr Saul's practice, I was used to making clinical decisions about treatments and initiating prescriptions for the GP to sign, and I agree with the statement in the Crown Report (DoH 1989):

> the nurse who plans and carries through a programme of care and has continuing contact with the patient is uniquely placed to make an accurate assessment of that patient's needs and is the person who should take responsibility for her decisions.
>
> (para 1.18, p. 17)

I started to prescribe on 4 of October 1994, and the benefits to me and to the patients were felt immediately.

Time-saving

Time is precious to nurses and patients alike. Not having to go backwards and forwards to the surgery or stand outside the doctor's room to get his signature saves both the doctor's and the nurse's time. Treatments are therefore commenced more quickly, giving a better service to the patients. An example of this is Mrs Brown (not her real name), who was discharged from hospital to a residential home on Friday afternoon. She was a diabetic, new to insulin. She was catheterised and was on twice daily insulin injections. I visited Mrs Brown at 5.00 p.m. to give her insulin injection and found that she had been discharged with just two insulin syringes and one night drainage bag. At 5.00 p.m. on Friday, this would have caused difficulties for the nurse, doctor and patient in trying to get the necessary equipment from the surgery to last over the weekend. I was able to prescribe the insulin syringes and the drainage bags immediately, with much relief on the part of the care staff and the patient, and saving time for all concerned.

Stockpiling

Prior to nurse prescribing, the delay in getting prescriptions would often lead to patients stockpiling dressings or other products for fear of 'running out'. I am now able to prescribe more appropriate amounts, and there is therefore less waste. It was nearly 12 months before I needed to prescribe a dressing pack for one lady on my caseload: she had 48 in stock, and we only used one dressing pack per week.

Better compliance

The nurse often has more time than the doctor to explain how to take medication or how to use a product, and this may lead to better compliance. I visited a 65-year-old gentleman who had suffered a cardiovascular accident and had been discharged from hospital 2 days previously. He had made a good recovery and had regained much of his independence. His main problem was pain in his affected arm, for which he was taking Co-dydramol, two tablets four times a day. One of the side-effects of these tablets is constipation, of which this gentleman was complaining. After advising about his diet, I also recommended an osmotic laxative, which he then said he had taken before without success. After deeper discussion, he revealed that he had taken one dose at night and had expected to have a bowel movement the following morning. When this did not happen, he had decided it was 'no good'. I prescribed the laxative and explained that it would take 48 hours to work and that he would need to drink extra fluids. He would need to take the laxative regularly for as long as he needed the analgesics. When this gentleman understood the reason for his constipation and how this could be overcome by taking the laxative properly, he complied with the treatment, and, by also including fruit and fibre in his diet, his problem was solved.

Cost awareness

As prescribers, we have definitely become more aware of costs, and, while the aim of the scheme is not to save money but to give a better service to patients and enhance the nurse's role (Cumberlege 1995), I felt that the cost implication would be a major issue in determining the success or failure of the pilot. By prescribing more appropriate amounts and cheaper products, where appropriate, we actually achieved a cost saving in Bolton.

Continuity of care

Nurse prescribing has improved the care given to our patients and families. Patients like continuity of care, and the nurse–patient relationship has improved. Consider, for example, Mrs Smith (not her real name), a 56-year-old lady with terminal cancer. She was very poorly and in the late stages of her illness. On visiting Mrs Smith on Sunday morning, I found that she had been very uncomfortable all night and had not passed urine for 24 hours. She had not wanted to call out the doctor as he had visited the day before and she feared it would be a 'rota doctor' who did not know her. On examination, her bladder was very distended, and she was obviously retaining urine. I phoned the doctor to discuss Mrs Smith's condition; he was quite happy for me to catheterise the patient. The prescription for the necessary items was written. Mr Smith went to the pharmacy while I was attending to his wife, and within 45 minutes Mrs Smith was catheterised, her relief being very satisfying to see. The continuity of care at this stage of Mrs Smith's illness was very important to her, and being able to identify the problem, plan, implement and evaluate the care, without needing a visit from a doctor whom she had never seen before, improved her sense of well-being. Other benefits could also be seen from this case: the time saved for the doctor, who did not need to visit just to prescribe the necessary equipment; for the nurse, who did not have to return to the patient after the doctor had visited; for the patient, who did not have to wait too long for the treatment to be commenced.

Health promotion

Noack (1987) defines health promotion as a personal approach to individual behaviour change in response to health education. Nurse prescribing has led to increased opportunities for health promotion, for example with regard to bowel management. Rather than prescribing a laxative, time will be taken to discuss diet and lifestyle, and, with encouragement and monitoring, a prescription is sometimes unnecessary. The only concern about nurse prescribing voiced by the doctors at our practice was with regard to the prescribing of laxatives and the fear that a serious condition could remain undetected. The team discussed this at length and agreed that good communication between nurses and doctors was vital. Since the start of nurse prescribing, communication has vastly improved, and the team has been strengthened because of it.

Health visitor

As a newly qualified health visitor, my anxieties initially centred around the actual writing of the prescription, although I was well aware that, as professionals, we initiate a wide range of treatments and prescriptions; my confidence in relation to nursing assessment and diagnosis seemed to diminish when I realised that I would be totally responsible for the episode of care when signing the prescription. I was conscious of the fact that it is not just the issue of prescribing, but also the professional accountability that goes with the prescribing, that is important. Although, in the past, I considered the ethical, legal and accountability issues when providing care for patients, I often did so subconsciously. One of the major professional benefits for me now is that I do consider all aspects of my duty of care, not just in relation to prescribing; also, through reflective practice, I re-evaluate a larger percentage of my professional roles and responsibilities. Murphy and Atkins (1994) define the reflective process, suggesting that:

> Because reflection involves exploration of a unique situation, new knowledge may be generated. Reflection therefore has the potential to address the problems of practice in a way that the application of technical rational approaches alone do not.
>
> (p.13)

It is hoped that, by presenting the following case studies (names have been changed to protect the identities of the clients and maintain confidentiality), the reader will be able to recognise reflection in practice, approaches to care and the professional autonomy that has been gained through nurse prescribing.

Working as part of the primary health care team has meant that communication has been greatly improved, especially between GPs, pharmacists and community nurses who are currently prescribing. This is re-affirmed by Luker *et al.* (1997) in the *Evaluation of Nurse Prescribing Final Report* (section 6.5). The focus of reflection is upon the analysis of practice situations to explain what is happening from the professional perspective.

Case study 1

Melissa, aged 2 months, attended the surgery for her primary course of immunisations. Carole, her mother, was very anxious regarding any possible side-effects. Melissa was Carole's first baby, and this was adding to her anxiety. Carole was a young single parent and doubted she would be able to cope in an emergency should there be any complications following immunisation.

Nursing actions and outcome

Descriptions of the vaccines offered were given to Carole, who decided that Melissa was to have oral polio and the combined injection of diphtheria, tetanus, pertussis and Hib.

Possible reactions to vaccines were carefully explained to Carole, and local reaction at the injection site and the possibility of systemic febrile illness were detailed. Any questions Carole asked were answered openly and honestly. Reassurance was given to Carole that not all babies suffer these reactions, and she was also advised to give paracetamol oral suspension to Melissa in the event of febrile illness. Carole asked if I could give her some paracetamol, so I wrote a prescription for paracetamol oral suspension, 2 ml to be given 6 hourly to a maximum of two doses.

I had established prior to vaccination that Melissa was well, had not had any previous injections and had never had any other treatment for any other conditions. I also explained to Carole the signs and symptoms she should look for if febrile illness occurred. The management of febrile illness was also discussed, for example tepid sponging, avoiding too much body contact and wearing cool cotton clothing. Carole was advised to use a syringe when administering the paracetamol. I supplied the syringe and also advised Carole to make a note of the time of administration and what to expect from the treatment: relief from pain and a lowering of temperature. Carole was also assured that, if she were worried about Melissa's condition or she did not feel that the baby's temperature was under control, despite using paracetamol and other management techniques, she should seek the advice of the GP. If Melissa were seen by the doctor, Carole was to show the doctor the medicine prescribed and also state what had already been administered and when. This would avoid any confusion if another prescription were given for paracetamol by any other name, for example Calpol. The medication prescribed was recorded in the GP records and the child health record. Verbal instructions on management were reinforced in writing by way of the parent-held record.

The result

Melissa had a slight temperature; Carole gave one dose of paracetamol suspension and no further treatment was required. I felt that, in prescribing the paracetamol, I had made the right clinical decision. I was advocating the use of the medication during the consultation. When asked whether I could supply it, I felt more confident knowing that Carole would have the recommended medication, dose and application to treat febrile illness should it occur.

Case study 2

Mrs Bates attended a local cytology clinic for which I am responsible. She was a 46-year-old lady who had attended for a routine smear. During the assessment and screening, she declared that she had had vaginal and anal itching for 18 months. Mrs Bates had been seen by the GP but was reluctant to describe her symptoms fully as the GP was male and she was embarrassed. No cause for the itching was determined, and the patient had used various over-the-counter creams to try to alleviate the itch. Mrs Bates was currently using Locan, which was proving ineffective in relieving symptoms, especially at night when the itching was disturbing her sleep.

Nursing actions

During the procedure of taking the smear, I noted the areas of skin excoriation around the vulva and anal area; there was no evidence of acute infection, but I observed that Mrs Bates had threadworms. Once the smear was completed, I asked her if she had had a urine test recently. This was to try to exclude diabetes as an underlying cause for the pruritus. She said that she had had two urine tests, both of which were normal. The patient was not currently taking any oral medication and had no irregular bowel symptoms. I explained to Mrs Bates that she had threadworms; this was done sensitively and Mrs Bates was reassured that they could be treated easily and effectively. There was no need to go back to the GP at this stage.

Treatment

Mrs Bates lived with her husband. I explained the cause and treatment of threadworms and advised that both Mr and Mrs

Bates should receive treatment. Both adults paid for prescriptions, and I therefore advised them to buy piperazine and senna powders over the counter. Having explained the cycle of transfer for thread-worms, Mrs Bates was also advised to wash her hands and scrub her finger nails prior to eating or preparing food, and always after using the toilet. I suggested that she have a bath in the mornings to remove any new eggs laid overnight. If the sole cause of the pruritus were threadworms, the symptoms should disappear following treatment. If the symptoms persisted, it was suggested that she consult the GP for further investigations.

Reflecting back on this consultation, I feel that my assessment, history-taking and diagnosis were within my remit as a competent practitioner. I also feel that the situation needed a sensitive approach to prevent causing the patient unnecessary distress. My decision not to prescribe was justified; I do not feel it would have been ethical to prescribe when an over-the-counter purchase was much cheaper. I did, however, give a detailed explanation of the usage of the medication and also the expected outcomes.

Case study 3

I had gone to do a primary visit for Josh, an 11-day-old baby. During the visit, his mother, Mrs Smith, sought my advice regarding Ben, her elder 3-year-old son, who had recently developed constipation. He had not had his bowels open for a week and was complaining of 'tummy ache'. Mrs Smith had purchased Ex-Lax over the counter, with which to treat Ben.

Nursing actions and evaluation

During the visit, I observed Ben to be a rather active little boy. He was eating his lunch at a small table in front of the television; he constantly left the table to play, watch television and talk to his mummy. At the end of the visit, his lunch was cold and only half eaten. He was given a cup of milk, which he drank immediately, and went to play again. I had a long discussion with his mum regarding how Ben had coped with the arrival of Josh. It became apparent that all Ben's routines, including bedtime and mealtimes, had been disrupted. Ben had also indicated that he wanted to wear nappies despite the fact that he had been dry for 6 months.

I advised Mrs Smith that the arrival of Josh would have some impact on Ben's behaviour and suggested that Ben may be 'withholding' and not feeling comfortable having his bowels open on the potty, especially if there have been many visitors of late. Mrs Smith said she had been urging Ben to stay on the potty until he had had his bowels open in order to avoid him soiling his pants. Having discussed appropriate management techniques, I advised Mrs Smith that Ex-Lax was too strong a laxative for Ben.

Treatment

I prescribed some lactulose, explaining to Mrs Smith that it was a non-stimulant laxative and less aggressive; I also advised the need for increased fluids. Mrs Smith was going to attempt to re-establish Ben's routines, especially at mealtimes. I advised Mrs Smith that, once the lactulose had taken effect, she should allow Ben to have his bowels open while wearing a nappy if he was more comfortable doing this, until the initial problem of constipation was resolved. I also advised her not to make Ben use the potty against his wishes: he needed to regain regular bowel habit and confidence.

I was to go back 1 week later to give breastfeeding support and reassess the plan of care and future management for Ben. In this situation, I did not just prescribe; working in partnership with Mrs Smith, we made joint decisions regarding future management. The immediate problem of constipation would hopefully be resolved with the prescription of lactulose. This also needed to be reinforced with future management of Ben's routines and dietary habits, in the hope that constipation does not recur.

Case study 4

Jonathan attended surgery with his mum for a routine child development assessment. He was 3 years old. During the assessment, I noted Jonathan frequently scratching his head. When I mentioned this to Mrs Jones, his mother, she said he had had head lice 2 weeks ago; she thought he had got them at nursery. I checked Jonathan's hair, and he was infested with live head lice. Mrs Jones reported that she had only treated Jonathan and not the other family members. She had purchased Full Marks shampoo over the counter at the time but could not afford to treat her daughter Kerry and herself.

Nursing actions and evaluation

I prescribed Carbaryl lotion, alcoholic 0.5 per cent, having checked with the local pharmacist that this was the currently recommended treatment. I issued three prescriptions for Mrs Jones, Jonathan and Kerry. None of the family suffered from asthma or eczema, so there were no contraindications to using an alcoholic solution. I advised Mrs Jones on the correct usage and to follow the written instructions carefully. The myths regarding head lice were dispelled, and management techniques to comple-ment medication were discussed with regard to the grooming techniques needed to prevent reinfestation. Mrs Jones was advised to inform the nursery and the school that she had effectively treated the children for head lice. If she needed any further help, she could contact me at the surgery or health centre.

Case study 5

Mrs Cotes attended the well-baby clinic with her 6-week-old daughter, Bethany. Discussion took place regarding Bethany's progress in relation to development and feeding. Mrs Cotes reported that Bethany was unsettled following some feeds, partic-ularly in the evenings. Bethany was taking 6 oz formula feeds. She tolerated the amount well; however, Mrs Cotes reported that Bethany cried in the evenings and was drawing her legs up. Colic was discussed, and we decided that the use of Infacol prior to feeds would be appropriate to complement management techniques. During the visit, I also noted that Bethany had oral thrush; the cause and management of the condition was explained to Mrs Cotes.

Treatment

Bethany needed a prescription for nystatin 100,000 units/ml and Infacol drops. As a nurse prescriber, I was able to provide a prescription for nystatin; however, due to the limited NPF, I was unable to prescribe the Infacol drops. This necessitated Mrs Cotes arranging to see her GP, resulting in an unnecessary consultation that delayed Bethany's treatment and was a waste of Mrs Cote's and the GP's time.

Summary

I hope that these case studies show how, in my position as a health visitor, prescribing has enhanced the opportunities for working in partnership with patients and clients in the effective treatment and management of the conditions described. Chayass (1992) stresses that working in partnership improves the holistic approach to care by allowing an equal sharing of power within the relationship.

Health promotion and compliance with treatment are likely to have been improved and consolidated by issuing a prescription or advising over-the-counter purchases. Hunt and Macleod (1987) believe that nurses should be the ones to give detailed information to patients on the benefits of new approaches.

Management techniques have been highlighted in all cases, which should improve effective treatment and prevent the need for unnecessary consultations with the GP, or repeat prescriptions because treatment has failed.

In each of the cases outlined, I feel I can justify my practice in relation to assessment, diagnosis and treatment. Doctors are taught to use a medical model to enable them to reach a diagnosis and provide treatment; however, as nurses, we are taught to use a nursing/social model. I believe that nurse prescribing allows us to combine the two, and thus the patient receives appropriate care – which may not always result in the issuing of a prescription – promoting a holistic approach to the delivery of care. There is evidence in literature that identifies the dissatisfaction many people experience when trying to communicate with doctors (Cartwright 1967, Gregory 1978). Byrne and Lang (1976) conclude, in their study, that over 60 per cent of doctors gather information, analyse and probe to fit the patient into a medically defined disease category. The patient's involvement in this process of diagnosis is limited. The doctor may make little or no attempt to see the patient's situation from his or her point of view.

I have found that there has been a definite increase in professional autonomy. This has improved teamwork and nurse–patient relationships, and has allowed me to work as an equal member of the primary health care team. As a prescriber, I am now more professionally aware of the safety, ethical and economical issues involved in prescribing and patient care delivery.

It is recognised by the majority of health visitors that there are some omissions from the NPF, the addition of which would benefit us in meeting the needs of clients within the home. Following the evaluation of the nurse prescribing pilot, these could be addressed.

I have no doubts that nurse prescribing has improved professional and client relationships, resulting in a more appropriate use of professional skills and the enhancement of patient care.

Prescribing difficulties

Nurse prescribing was not without a few problems, the main one, initially, being the generic prescribing of wound care products. Having to write 'Vapour Permeable Adhesive Film Dressing' instead of 'OP Site' or 'Tegaderm' was impractical and time-consuming. Pharmacists were having great problems with these prescriptions and needed to know which specific brands were wanted. Fortunately, since April 1997, it has been acceptable to use brand names for wound care products, which has saved time for nurses and helped the pharmacists tremendously.

Another problem was record-keeping: having to record everything prescribed in three different places, that is, patient-held records, the GP's records and nurse records at the health centre, was time-consuming and, for some items, seemed unnecessary.

This was overcome following discussion with the Trust and the GPs. The decision was made that systemic medication was to be recorded on GP records as soon as possible but that wound care products and appliances needed only to be recorded on patient-held records, which are accessible to all health care professionals.

Extension to the original pilot

The evidence gleaned from the eight pilot sites was not considered to comprise sufficient data to generalise. The pilot sites only consisted of one GP practice in each of the regions, so the decision was made to extend the pilot to include a larger area. We were very pleased that Bolton was chosen, and, in April 1996, 120 nurses were trained to prescribe. When this news was announced, media attention began all over again and we were once more asked to give interviews and talks. This time, we were more prepared, having been prescribing for 18 months; we felt much more confident in answering questions.

All the GP practices in Bolton were taking part so we could now treat all our patients the same. When working in a clinic setting, it had become quite frustrating only being able to prescribe for Dr Saul's patients. We could now prescribe for any patient with a Bolton GP by writing the appropriate GP's code on the prescription form. Also, in the residential homes, where the residents have different GPs, it was much more convenient being able to prescribe for all our residential patients.

Conclusion

There is no doubt that nurse prescribing is a success in Bolton. All the community staff involved have commented on the improvement to patient care delivery that nurse prescribing has made. Nurses have proved that they can prescribe cost-effectively. The time-saving, continuity of care, better compliance and opportunities for health promotion are ensuring a more responsive and efficient service to our patients and clients. Prescribing has improved both job satisfaction and professional autonomy for the nurses involved.

Our goal must be to ensure, eventually, that every nurse in the country who is suitably trained and who is committed to nurse prescribing should be allowed to do so, in the interests of patients and the nursing profession.

(Cumberlege 1997)

As nurse prescribers, we hope that this comes to fruition sooner rather than later, enabling other nurses to experience the professional benefits that prescribing brings. Being involved in this major advance for community nurses has certainly increased our job satisfaction, and it is very rewarding to hear our colleagues say, 'What on earth did we do before?'

References

Byrne, P. and Lang, B. (1976) *Doctors Talking to Patients*. HMSO, London.

Carlisle, D (1989) Prescribing charge. *Community Outlook* November: p. 26.

Cartwright, A. (1967) *Patients and their Doctors*. Routledge, London.

Chayass, J. (1992) New dimensions of experiments in nursing. *Journal of Advanced Nursing* **17**: 1–2.

Cumberlege, J. (1995) Sharing prescribing power. *Community Nursing* **1**(1): 3.

Cumberlege, J. (1997) Nurse prescribing must not be for trading. *Nurse Prescribing Newsletter* **5**: 1.

DoH (1989) *Report of the Advisory Group on Nurse Prescribing*, p. 17 (Crown Report). DoH, London.

Gregory, J. (1978) Patients' attitudes to the hospital service. A survey resource paper (No.5). HMSO, London.

Hunt, J. (1988) Primary nursing the next challenge. *Nursing Times* **84**(49): 36, 38.

Hunt, S.M. and Macleod, M. (1987) Health and behavioural change: some lay perspectives. *Community Medicine* **9**(1): 68–76.

Luker, K.A., Austin, L., Hogg, C. *et al.* (1997) Evaluation of Nurse Prescribing Final Report: Executive Summary. Unpublished report.

Noack, H. (1987) *Concepts of Health Promotions: Measurement in Health Promotion and Protection*. WHO, Copenhagen.

Murphy, K. and Atkins, S. (1994) Reflection with a practice-led curriculum. In Palmer, A., Burns, S. and Bulman, C. (eds) *Reflective Practice in Nursing*, pp. 10–19. Blackwell Science, Oxford.

Pearson, A. (1987) *Nursing Quality Measurement: Quality Assurance Methods for Peer Review*. John Wiley & Sons, Chichester.

Tingle, J.H. (1990) Nurses and the law. *Nursing Times* **86**(38): 70–2.

Tschudin, V. (1986) *Ethics in Nursing*. Heinemann, London.

8   Do not go gentle...

David Skidmore

Dylan Thomas wrote a poem that begs one not meekly to accept death but to rage 'against the dying of the light' (Thomas 1987). Nurses, it seems, have to 'rage' in order to develop their role. Green indicates (Chapter 1) that nurse prescribing is not a new idea, having been mooted some 14 years before the first demonstration sites were announced. The demonstration was running for some 4 years prior to being rolled out to the district nursing and health visitor branches of community nursing. The exclusion of other community nurses makes a significant contribution to the secularisation of nursing.

The practitioner debate categorises nurses in terms of core, specialist and advanced. Core practice, it is suggested, is demonstrated by those skills achieved by way of first-level registration and equips nurses to undertake generalist activities (Poulton 1997). The specialist practitioner should demonstrate higher levels of practice; this will involve study at degree level (UKCC 1994). The advanced practitioner is still ill defined (UKCC 1996). However, Woods (1998) argues that those nurses who undertake advanced practitioner courses experience difficulty in describing their role. Furthermore, they tend to find themselves somewhat alienated from nursing colleagues. It is argued that elevating the status of practice is more than the sum total of courses completed and, if measured only by the level of academic achievement, may be disruptive within a nursing culture. Nurse prescribing could be seen to elevate the practice of an exclusive group of nurses, a group who belong to those categorised as specialist practitioners.

Groves (Chapter 2) argues that nursing has advanced considerably in terms of autonomy and practice; I would argue that much of that advancement has taken place at a rapid pace from the 1980s onward. However, such advancement is not uniform in terms of recognition, and it seems contradictory to recognise all community nurses as specialist practitioners and yet limit nurse prescribing to just two groups. Such limitation has serious implications for the realisation of effective teamwork and a 'seamless' service. Groves quite rightly suggests that nurse prescribing can only be beneficial for the advancement of nursing practice and yet, in terms of its introduction, it may be divisive.

The early 1990s held the promise of a new horizon for nursing: one voice, a voice that would take nursing forward. There really was a possibility that nurses would come together as a unified body. Unfortunately, the further development of educational programmes now seems to militate against such unification. The titles 'specialist' and 'advanced' suggest skills beyond those practised by the everyday, common or garden nurse. Indeed, the UKCC (1994) states that the specialist will demonstrate the development of practice through research, improve standards of care through supervised practice and demonstrate higher levels of decision-making. This higher level of practice can only be accessed after first-level registration. Does this suggest, then, that the first-level nurse, with her core skills, is a lesser nurse? Should she forget the art of nursing that is embedded in caring and concentrate on those skills which can claim higher qualifications? Caring, the essence of nursing, is very difficult to assess in the academic sense; peers, however, often have an accurate view of what makes a good nurse. Therein lies the rub. If legislation grants more autonomy to one group of nurses, there is an inequality that prevents effective peer review.

The present nurse prescribers' course (1994–98) is only open to health visitors and district nurses (or practice nurses who hold either qualification). This suggests that these nurses already possess some unique skill or knowledge that places them apart from 'ordinary' nurses. Oddly, Poulton (1997) suggests that it is practice nurses who hold a more generic role in primary health, and yet, unless they hold the HV or DN qualification, they are ineligible for nurse prescriber courses even though they are (from 1997) recognised as specialist practitioners. Green (Chapter 1) argues that nurse prescribing is a major step forward for nursing and Groves (Chapter 2) that it will help to reduce the hours that junior doctors are required to work. I would, however, stress Green's comment that we should hope that the current situation is only the beginning. To be of real benefit to the health service (in its fiftieth year), nurse prescribing must be extended to at least all specialist practitioner nurses.

There are thousands of practice nurses who will be denied the right to prescribe, and Poulton (1997) reveals that there has been a 300 per cent increase in the number of practice nurses employed in general practice. Indeed, the intensive interest in practice nursing (Poulton 1997) suggests that they will be the key workers in community health by the millennium. The situation created by nurse prescribing within practice nursing illuminates the future implications for nursing as a whole. In the demonstration sites, the situation exists whereby a small number of practice nurses can prescribe but a larger number cannot. The licence to prescribe sets a minority of practice nurses apart from their colleagues. There is one school of thought arguing that practice nurses have always prescribed; but the practice that they put forward as evidence is not autonomous practice and is also illegal. Nurse prescribers, on the other hand, have government blessing to possess a skill denied to others in their ranks.

Woods (1998) argues that such practices alienate nurses from their colleagues because they are viewed in a different way. The practice and everyday demeanour of the nurses may not change, yet others will perceive them as having changed. Nurse prescribers can maintain their behaviour in a fashion identical to that of their colleagues but need only sign one prescription to be confirmed as different. Mental health nursing offers evidence of how this might develop in practice.

During the 1970s, in the field of psychiatry, two groups of nurses became similarly isolated: community psychiatric nurses and, what were then, behavioural therapists. They were accused of not wanting to be nurses any more, of being mental health visitors or 'wannabe' psychologists. The subsequent alienation led to the formation of their own associations or their joining more welcoming groups (the British Association of Behavioural Psychotherapy), thereby confirming to on-lookers that they were trying to be more than a nurse. In truth, these groups were looking for mutual support to help them to cope with new nursing developments (Skidmore and Friend 1984). In practice, they unwittingly contributed to the secularisation of psychiatric nursing (Skidmore 1997). The solidarity of psychiatric nurses witnessed during the 1950s and 60s was rapidly becoming a thing of the past. In response to the Community Psychiatric Nurses Association, non-community psychiatric nurses formed the Psychiatric Nurses Association, and, although both groups stopped short of membership monopoly (that is, only permitting membership of one association, as in the rules of the medical Royal Colleges of the nineteenth century), great rivalries existed. One can speculate on how much more secure the future of psychiatric nursing would be today had the solidarity survived. Mental health nursing is on the verge of a manpower crisis within the next 10 years (Journal of Health Service Management 1997): there has not been the right level of recruitment and retention to offset the impending retirements.

Back to nurse prescribing, although the above diatribe is pertinent. Any separation of one nursing group will erode the common identity. It does not take a Marx or Durkheim to theorise about this: the evidence is in our own history. The grading exercise is one classic example. Community nurses during the 1980s were automatically graded G (or sister grade) even though they were novice community nurses. Did this not declare to the nursing world that they were superior to 'ordinary' ward nurses? The novice ward nurse had to be content with a D or E grade. Such grading issues create boundaries within the nursing culture that are indefensible. Certainly, being no altruist and having bills to pay, I, like so many others, was not going to refuse my charge nurse grade when I became a community nurse. I had taken extra responsibility, did not have the back-up of a nursing team and basically did not know what I was doing for a full 6 months; I was not unique (Skidmore and Friend 1984). The argument against allowing only the few into nurse prescribing is even more basic. What is so special about health visitors and district nurses that places them in a unique position whereby prescribing licences can be conferred upon them? The NHS Executive (1996) claims that the health visitor role is focused on the wider public health agenda whereas:

> district nurses address clearly defined health needs, largely with the housebound and elderly.

While I can see the rationale for including district nurses in the prescribing team, I cannot justify the inclusion of health visitors. I do not seek to denigrate health visiting but view the health visitor's role in a more proactive sense; they are truly in the front line of prevention, for which there are few, if any, prescriptions. It could be argued that they have moved out of nursing *per se*; in fact, it is only with the new specialist community awards that 'nursing' has crept back into the title. Indeed, there is now talk of locating health visitors under Home Office control (*Nursing Times* 1998). Singling out one group of nurses in this way is, of course, unfair; they, like any qualified nurses, should be allowed to prescribe. Please note the 'any qualified nurses'. When nurse prescribing rolls out, nursing is going to enter an *Animal Farm*-type phase:

All nurses are equal
but some nurses are more
equal than others.

(after Orwell 1945)

Nurse prescribing can only be good for nursing. Green (Chapter 1) argues that it is seen as a valuable component of community nursing. It could be so much more in terms of unifying nursing. In the midst of confusion on the part of the professional boards with regard to what specialist practice is (*Nursing Times* 1997), the profession is still willing to confer an aegis of speciality on certain groups. While there is dissent, (Jones and Gough 1997), the professional body appears to be going 'gentle into that good night'. The major outcome will be that these two groups will be more specialist than the other specialist practitioners since only two of the eight specialist community branches will be allowed to prescribe. Since the UKCC decided in March 1997 not to establish explicit standards for advanced practice, it is difficult to know how to locate this élite workforce. It will certainly add to the confusion of attempting to define specialist practitioners.

Castledine (quoted in Mahoney 1997) argues that specialist practitioner status is reflected in clinical skill rather than courses completed, and that it is practice led rather than education led. Unfortunately, his argument, while being laudable, is not supported by that which is actually happening. Consider nurse prescribing as a practitioner skill. Quite rightly, it should be assessed through practice: only then can it be practice led. It is currently indeed a reflection of courses completed: health visiting or district nursing plus nurse prescribers' course equals super-specialist practitioner. One could also question whether or not the current arrangements to become a community specialist practitioner are practice led. Nurses must still complete a recognised course; demonstration of experience and clinical skill is not sufficient. Practice nurses can certainly submit evidence to recognised centres to be 'upgraded' to specialist practitioner level, and paediatric community nurses will shortly have the same opportunity; nevertheless, upgrading will depend on the number of courses that the nurse has completed. Castledine (quoted in Mahoney 1997, p. 8) goes on to suggest that:

> We have got to develop a framework for evaluation or the term [specialist practitioner] could fall into disrepute.

Given that more balls are thrown into the juggling act (almost every week it seems), forming committees to develop such frameworks is rather futile. There is now a call for nurse anaesthetists (Audit Commission 1997); where will these fit into the specialist versus advanced debate? All the committees in the world are doomed to failure when trying to unravel this Gordian knot of nursing since they have yet to define and agree just what a nurse is. Nurse prescribing adds more strands to the knot in that it is reserved for an élite group of nurses. It should, however, be a basic skill of all first-level nurses. After all, the formulary is hardly earth-shatteringly dangerous; patients are not going to die from an overprescription of dressings... so why are the DoH and the professional bodies so cautious in its introduction? Added to this conundrum is the fact that one of the groups entitled to enter nurse prescribing courses (health visitors) is under threat nationwide. Throughout November and December 1997, the *Nursing Times* carried news reports of massive redundancies in health visiting. Add the point that nurses should take over half of the GP's workload (Nuffield Trust 1997) and the knot becomes tighter and more difficult to untie. Obviously, if nurses are to take on some of the functions of GPs, they must prescribe; yet the nurse whose role is closest to that of the GP is currently disqualified from entering the prescribers' course.

The starting point to this debate is that all qualified nurses should be licensed to prescribe. This is the only tenet that will recognise all nurses as equal. It is also the only starting point that will permit sense to be made of specialist and advanced practitioners, especially if one accepts that such titles are won through a practice-led framework. A staged recognition of basic practical skills (and prescribing is a basic skill) cannot work. Imagine the newly qualified medical doctor who has to refer a patient to a colleague for a prescription! It is quite ludicrous.

There is, however, a negative aspect contained in the process of rolling out nurse prescribing to all nurses: it will undoubtedly add to the blurring of doctor–nurse roles. Giving added responsibility to nurses, in whatever environment, has the consequence of nurses having to prioritise their duties. Some activities will be seen as being of less importance, with the result that some nursing skills will be marginalised. The greatest danger is that prescribing will form a barrier to nurse–patient communication. In the past, the nurse was seen as a carer, and this facilitated communication with patients. The new role will change the way in which nurses are seen by the public. They will, indeed, become demi-gods in the way that doctors are gods. Obviously, this will not be a deliberate act on the part of the nurse, but the fact that nurses have a legal right to prescribe suggests that they have more power than the average nurse.

Nurse prescribing is not necessarily a bad thing, although its introduction could be devastating for nursing. There is a lot to lose, the art and practice of nursing being paramount. If nurse prescribing must be introduced, all qualified nurses should be allowed to prescribe... but let nurses beware of the consequences. One only has to recall the fate of theatre nurses to recognise the implications. Theatre nurses are no longer required because theatre technicians exist. Nurses rarely take blood samples now because phlebotomists have been created. Bed-making has also become a back page of nursing history. If nurses are not careful, some future historian could well be asking, where did all the nurses go? There is an aggressive movement to institute doctors' assistants, and many nurses support this. Nurse prescribing facilitates this new identity of the hybrid nurse, casting off the mantle of nursing and taking on the partial cloak of the doctor. On the positive side, it could render the specialist practitioner debate redundant; on the negative side, it could signal the death knell of nursing as we know it in the UK.

Nurse prescribing could have been used to help to define primary health care nursing. Although it has been argued that it should be accessible by all qualified nurses, it has in reality been conferred on the few; had it been thought through, it could have unified nursing practice in primary health. There is a need to revisit the issue of what is required in primary health nursing, but that need not exclude health visitors and district nurses. It should certainly not require the replacement of nurses with assistant doctors. Nurses are nurses; if they lose sight of that fact, the whole arena of health care becomes a circus. The proposed roll-out of nurse prescribing may, in its present form, be divisive for nurses. All qualified nurses possess the experience and ability to prescribe. Nursing is essentially a practitioner role; it should, indeed, be practice led. Nurse prescribing is a part of practice rather than a right to be claimed by having done the right courses. While it is logical that nurses prescribe, it is criminal that nursing is fragmented by limiting nurse prescribing.

The benefits of extending the role of the 'nurse' (archaic term) cannot be denied. It will offer more accessibility to the patient, save doctors' time and be economically sound. All of this is good. What is not understandable is why only a small proportion of nurses are being given prescribing rights when the argument for giving all nurses prescribing powers is so sound. It has been mentioned above that the NPF will hardly be life-threatening if abused. Why not, then, extend this to all qualified nurses?

There is a precarious future for nursing if nurse prescribing is to be confined to élite groups. It transcends the specialist practitioner debate in that it clearly identifies a group of nurses who have 'higher' skills than the rest. Nurse prescribing has been educationally led and there has been little objection from practitioners; this does not bode well for the future of nursing. The professional bodies have been complacent about the form of assessment for nurse prescribing: a classroom-based examination. The educationalists involved in the pilot scheme wanted a practical aspect to the examination but were overruled – hardly a practice-led venture!

It would seem that the future of community nursing has been identified. It lies with the practice nurse (who is currently being upgraded to specialist practitioner). The evidence is offered by the DoH in the publication *Practice Nursing: A Changing Role to Meet Changing Needs* (Poulton 1997). A major role for the practice nurse is seen as health maintenance, including the management of conditions such as:

● asthma, diabetes and hypertension

the monitoring of:

● epilepsy, arthritis, anaemia, coronary heart disease and mental illness

and the treatment or management of:

● leg ulcers, wounds and eating disorders

– all conditions that could eventually lead to an extension of the NPF. How can it be, then, that the very nurses identified by Poulton (1997) as being in the front line of primary care are excluded from nurse prescribing courses? (Only 14 per cent of practice nurses have a recognised community nursing qualification.) Come to think of it, how does one recognise a community nursing qualification?

So what implication does nurse prescribing have for the future of nursing? Unfortunately, there is no simple answer: it really does depend upon how nurses receive it. It could be the saviour or equally the executioner of nursing. It could provide a starting point for basic nursing skills and, subsequently, explain specialist and advanced practitioners. It will certainly be divisive unless all qualified nurses can prescribe.

References

Audit Commission (1997) *Anaesthesia Under Examination*. Audit Commission, London.

Jones, M. and Gough, P. (1997) Nurse prescribing – why has it taken so long? *Nursing Standard* 11(20): 39–42.

Journal of Health Service Management (1997). News. **107**(5542): 7.

Mahoney, C. (1997) Bid to end confusion over specialist practice. *Nursing Times* **93**(50): 8.

NHS Executive (1996) *Primary Care: The Future*. NHSE, Leeds.

Nuffield Trust (1997) *The Physician Workforce in the UK*. Nuffield Trust, London.

Nursing Times (1998). This Week. *Nursing Times* **94**(27): 5.

Orwell, G. (1945) *Animal Farm*. Secker & Warburg, London.

Poulton, B. (1997) *Practice Nursing: A Changing Role to Meet Changing Needs*. DoH, London.

Skidmore, D. (1997) The Decline of the British Nurse. Third International Conference, Martin, Slovakia.

Skidmore, D. and Friend, W. (1984) Muddling through. *Nursing Times*: *Community Outlook*. 9 May, pp. 179–81.

Thomas, D. (1987) Do not go gently into that good night. In Wain, J. (ed.) *Oxford Library of English Poetry*. Oxford University Press, Oxford.

UKCC (1994) *The Council's Standards for Education and Practice following Registration*. Registrar's Letter. UKCC, London.

UKCC (1996) PREP: *The Nature of Advanced Practice*. CC/96146. UKCC, London.

Woods, L. (1998) Reconstructing nursing: a study of role transition in advanced nursing practice. Unpublished PhD thesis. Keele University.

9 Nurse prescribing: the future

Jennifer Humphries and Joyce Green

This final chapter of the book will look forward to examine nurse prescribing as it becomes part of community nursing practice not just for a few, but for many thousands of nurses who work in the community.

In April 1998, the Health Secretary, Frank Dobson, announced a national roll-out of community nurse prescribing. Fourteen million pounds is available, which Mr Dobson has said is a symbol of the government's commitment to nursing (Coombes and Porter 1998). The plan is to train 20,000 community nurses and health visitors, and Gulland (1998) reported that Mr Dobson has pledged to extend prescribing to other specialist nurses, with as many as 60,000 becoming prescribers. The money allocated to the health authorities, which will be available from September 1998, will buy the education programmes and provide replacement cover for staff during their training. It is also intended to help them to set up the infrastructure to support nurse prescribing (Sackman 1998).

At the present time, it is a topic for speculation whether or not the final report from the review committee chaired by Dr June Crown will recommend that the capacity to prescribe be granted to other community specialist practitioner branches or groups of nurses. At the time of writing, it appears that no nursing group has been ruled in, or out, of the scheme (*Nursing Times* 1998). While all community practitioner specialities are likely to be able to see benefits for their particular client group if prescribing is extended, there is clearly some way to go in terms of what may be prescribed by nurses and in what circumstances. Under current legislation, only those community nurses with a health visitor or district nurse qualification are permitted to attend courses to become nurse prescribers. There are other nursing groups, such as nurse practitioners and nurses with a specialist role, for example stoma therapists, diabetic specialist nurses and family planning nurses, who would also like to be given this opportunity. Should this happen, there will be implications for education and training and the development of the NPF which is presently considered restrictive by some current nurse prescribers.

Current nursing developments in community and primary health care

The NHS (Primary Care) Act 1997 has resulted in 10 nurse-led pilot sites, including some that are part of the nurse prescribing initiative (Queens Nursing Institute 1998). With the proposals presented in the new NHS White Paper (DoH 1997), the role of community nurses has been given a higher profile, and, according to Ballard (1998), 'the government believes that involving front-line clinicians, both family doctors and community nurses, is a solution to providing better care for patients'. Ballard points out that 'In this context, the term "community nurse" is used to include all nurses who work in the primary and community health sector'. Community NHS trusts are asked actively to facilitate the involvement of community nursing staff in local discussions on the establishment and development of primary care groups. Practice nurses should also be encouraged to participate. The primary care group will be looking at ways of improving the health of the population it serves. This will naturally include issues relating to the effectiveness and efficiency of the care provided, and the role of nurses in prescribing is likely to deliberated.

Nurse practitioners and clinical nurse specialists

Nurse practitioners and some types of clinical nurse specialist are keen to become prescribers. This would seem to be a natural progression from the work they are already doing; for example, many are prescribing under protocols. It should be emphasised that 'Group protocols are not about prescribing, but rather they are to enable nurses to supply and administer medication' (Sackman 1998). For many nurse practitioners and clinical nurse specialists, this arrangement for patient medication may be more suitable than nurse prescribing. However there may be others who find this method restrictive.

Developing nurse prescribing to become an integral part of the nurse practitioner role would seem pertinent when the UK role definition of the nurse practitioner is presented:

> The RCN Institute of Advanced Nurse Education (IANE) sees the nurse practitioner in primary health care as offering a complementary service to that of the general medical practitioner, offering 'direct access to clients seeking health care', and being able to 'undertake clinical assessments of any health problems likely to be encountered' and 'initiate treatment falling within her range of knowledge and skills'.
>
> (Jones 1996, p. 302)

Not all clinical nurse specialists will consider nurse prescribing relevant to their role. Nursing specialists function in a wide variety of specialist areas, and there is a disparity of practice even within the same, or a similar, field of speciality (Willis 1998). Nevertheless, Willis (1998) points out that the clinical nurse specialist should take opportunities to study for relevant courses. In the future, it may be that a nurse prescribing course would fulfil this requirement for some nurses working in certain specialist arenas.

Group protocols

One of the most controversial issues associated with nurse prescribing has been the widespread use of group protocols:

> A group protocol is a specific instruction for the supply and administration of named medicines in a clinical situation. It is drawn up locally by doctors, pharmacists and other appropriate professionals, and approved by employers, who are advised by the relevant professional advisory committees. It applies to groups of patients or other service users who may not be individually identified before presentation for treatment.
>
> (Cresswell 1998)

Nurses who have been working in the grey area of supplying and administering medicines under group protocols will have welcomed the publication of the interim Crown review at the end of April 1998 (DoH 1998) as much of the uncertainty surrounding the usage of these protocols has been lifted. Although the review does not clear up the legal ambiguities, it does recommend that the legal position be clarified to ensure that health professionals are acting legally. Health Secretary Frank Dobson, in responding to this recommendation, pledged that his department would address any ambiguities in the law for health professionals using group protocols. The review team recommended that current safe practice should continue until the legislation has been changed.

By analysing current practice, the review team found that standards varied and lines of accountability and responsibility were not always clear and documented. Group protocols tended to be used for the provision of contraceptive services and public health programmes, and in secondary care situations (Cresswell 1998). The report has provided health professionals with specific guidelines for drawing up group protocols, which should include clear statements regarding:

- the clinical situation to which the protocol applies
- the staff authorised to take responsibility for the supply or administration of medicines under a group protocol
- the description of treatment available under a group protocol.

According to Cresswell (1998), community nurses now have a framework to protect themselves and their patients and need to ensure that the group protocols they are working under comply with the stated criteria of the report. Although, as stated in the recommendation of the report, it is anticipated that most patients should continue to receive medicines on an individual basis as part of a comprehensive health service, there is likely to be a need for group protocols in certain limited situations.

Education and training

The education and training required to enable nurses to prescribe safely and effectively must continue to be carefully monitored. It is likely that pre-registration courses will incorporate more pharmacology and diagnostic skills that will prepare nurses for specialist roles in the future. At the time of writing, the transitional arrangements made by the UKCC (1996) are applicable to nurse prescribing; there are those who are able to use the title 'specialist practitioner' and those who have achieved the specialist qualification. The latter can only be gained on completion of a course approved by the ENB satisfying the UKCC (1995) criteria that include degree level study. From 1998, all academic institutions providing specialist community qualifications in any of the eight areas of practice must do so at this level. This course is intensive, and incorporating nurse prescribing into an already packed programme will require careful consideration by the educational institutions offering specialist community practitioner awards. The course will need to include a module that specifically addresses prescribing; this could be arranged in the common core framework if all or most of the eight branches were involved in future prescribing. However, as prescribing becomes the norm for the different community specialist practitioners, it will also need to be fully integrated into all aspects of the course and will therefore be covered within specialist modules as well.

For those community nurses who already had a post-registration clinical qualification relevant to their practice, gaining the nurse prescribing qualification will be likely to follow the format currently used by the demonstration site nurses. Health visitors, district nurses and practice nurses with either of those qualifications can probably feel confident that they will be included in the roll-out since the benefits of prescribing within their sphere of practice have been demonstrated.

When and how other specialist nurses will become involved is speculative at present, although the principles of shared learning currently employed in the education and training would apply no matter what specialities were included. The original ENB (1994) Open Learning Pack has been revised; although the content remains largely untouched from the original, the format is more user friendly. Practitioners will continue to be encouraged to work with colleagues, and it is essential that support from employers enables the students to work competently through the learning experiences.

Once qualified as a nurse prescriber, the same conditions that currently apply to those using the title 'specialist practitioner' have to continue to be met within the new realm of practice. Thus the practitioner and the employer must be confident that the practitioner has the skills and knowledge to fulfil his or her role effectively, taking the *Scope of Professional Practice* (UKCC 1992a) and the *Code of Professional Conduct* (UKCC 1992b) into account (Wallace 1998).

Current issues for consideration

Prescribing is a new venture for nurses and will naturally raise questions and concerns from members of the profession. The pioneers of the nurse prescribing initiative did not enter into the venture lightly. In an interview in 1996, Baroness Cumberlege said:

> My great passion has been nurse prescribing, I have been with it for ten years and I am determined it will succeed. But I have to be very careful that it doesn't fall apart, which it might if we haven't got the proper systems in place; if we haven't got the appropriate training; if the formulary is wrong; or if nurses actually feel inadequate. I would rather build on solid foundations and see the scheme succeed.
>
> (Williams 1996, p. 22)

The nurse prescribing pilot was evaluated by a highly qualified and competent team led by Professor Karen Luker, a renowned expert in the fields of both community nursing and research. The nursing profession is fortunate in having such members and that the validity and reliability of findings are open to scrutiny for all interested parties. If the DoH can be comfortable with the results of the pilot and demonstration nurse prescribing initiatives, nurses should feel reassured that the benefits of their prescribing are in the best interests of their patients and their own professional practice.

Nonetheless, change of any description can cause anxiety, and while there are many nurses who will embrace the venture wholeheartedly, there are bound to be those with reservations. Some (although very few) of the now-qualified nurse prescribers had more than the natural concerns that might be expected to occur with any new professional undertaking. The training is intended to equip nurses with the knowledge and skills necessary to be able to prescribe from the current NPF. Practical and theoretical education goes a long way to assuaging anxieties, although the original prescribers deserve recognition for taking the nursing profession forward into an unknown arena. These nurses were chosen carefully; they were known to have supportive mechanisms in place, including a properly functioning primary health care team and a responsive management structure. Nevertheless, the initial training of a 2-day residential course, including the examination, was criticised by the nurses as being too intensive and was subsequently changed to 3 separate days over 2 weeks, the examination taking place the following week. Interestingly, the apprehension over the examination appeared to be greater than over the prescribing in practice. Since most people are likely to face examinations with some trepidation, this cannot be viewed as reflecting a practitioner's ability to prescribe. In addition to the evaluation study conducted by Luker *et al.* (1997), the nursing press has produced some information about how the pilot and demonstration site nurses are faring in their role as prescribers (Alderman 1996, Smith 1996, Winstanley 1996, Blatt 1997, Carlisle 1997). The overwhelming view is positive, suggesting that, for these early prescribers, prescribing in practice appears to have caused little anxiety. As more nurses become prescribers, they have additional support in colleagues who are already prescribing, and, as the programme rolls out to involve more of the profession, it would seem pertinent to formalise this provision. It is likely that, with more nurses becoming prescribers, concerns will lessen as new prescribers become familiar with the role before becoming prescribers themselves.

Clearly, the nursing profession cannot be complacent; those with reservations about nurse prescribing undoubtedly have genuine reasons for their apprehension. It would not be prudent to dismiss these, and even staunch proponents of the scheme would do well to listen and respond to any misgivings that appear. So far, little evidence is available to indicate the level or type of doubt that exists within nursing. This may be because many nurses not directly involved with the project have only slight information on which to base an informed argument. Moreover, reading about nurse prescribing is not the same as practising as a prescriber. Current prescribers who experience problems should be able to address these within existing frameworks in their own area of practice. Nurses are perhaps more reticent in sharing examples of poor practice with a larger audience of peers than they would be in the relative safety of a small primary health care team meeting or clinical supervision session. In addition the generally positive atmosphere that surrounds nurse prescribing can perhaps deter those unsure of its benefits from venturing a less favourable opinion. Those of us convinced of the benefits for the nursing profession, and importantly for patient and client care, need to create a climate in which honest opinion can be aired. There is a clear need for regular evaluation and the reporting of both positive and not so positive issues that arise within the arena of nurse prescribing. While anecdotal information is useful, the importance of properly structured and organised research cannot be overestimated. The new NHS White Paper (DoH 1997) is committed to providing national standards and guidelines, and emphasises the importance of clinical and cost-effectiveness based on scientific evidence. Nurse prescribers have a responsibility to share their knowledge and skills to ensure that the quality of the nurse prescribing initiative maintains its momentum.

References

Alderman, C. (1996) Prescribing pioneers. *Nursing Standard* **10**(18): 26–7.

Ballard, H. (1998) The new NHS – modern and dependable. *Nursing Care, Journal of Community and District Nursing* Spring: 4–6.

Blatt, B. (1997) Nurse prescribing: are you ready? *Practice Nursing* **8**(12): 11–13.

Carlisle, D. (1997) Nurse prescribing wound dressings. *Nursing Times* **93**(28): 58–61.

Coombes, R. and Porter, R. (1998) Prescribing gets £14m boost. *Nursing Times* **94**(16): 5.

Cresswell, J. (1998) Group protocols and the law. *Community Nurse* **4**(5): 37–9.

DoH (1997) *The New NHS: Modern, Dependable. Executive Summary.* DoH, London.

DoH (1998) *Review of Prescribing, Supply and Administration of Medicines: A Report on the Supply and Administration Under Group Protocols.* DoH, London.

ENB (1994) *Nurse Prescribing Open Learning Pack.* ENB, London.

Gulland, A. (1998) The paperchase. *Nursing Times* **94**(17): 17.

Jones, M. (1996) The nurse practitioner in the community. In Gastrell, P. and Edwards, J. (eds) *Community Health Nursing: Frameworks for Practice.* Baillière Tindall/RCN, London.

Luker, K.A., Austin, L., Hogg, C. *et al.* (1997) Evaluation of Nurse Prescribing Final Report: Executive Summary. Unpublished report.

Nursing Times (1998) This Week. *Nursing Times* **94**(25): 9.

Queens Nursing Institute (1998) Go-ahead for first nurse-led pilot sites. *Newsletter* **8**(1): 4–5.

Sackman, T. (1998) Prescribed treatment. *Community Practitioner* **71**(7/8): 243.

Smith, K. (1996) Prescriptions in a different hand. *Community Nurse* **2**(7): 8.

UKCC (1992a) *Scope of Professional Practice*. UKCC, London.

UKCC (1992b) *Code of Professional Practice*. UKCC, London.

UKCC (1995) *The Future of Professional Practice. The Council's Standards for Education and Practice Following Registration (PREP)*. Position Statement (No. 2). UKCC, London.

UKCC (1996) *The Future of Professional Practice. The Council's Standards for Education and Practice Following Registration (PREP). Transitional Arrangements – Specialist Practitioner Title/Specialist Qualification*. Registrars Letter 15. UKCC, London.

Wallace, M. (1998) Specialist practice: the transitional arrangements. *Nursing Times Learning Curve* **2**(3): 2–3.

Williams, K. (1996) Convinced of the cause. *Nursing Standard* **10**(23): 22–3.

Willis, J. (1998) The clinical nurse specialist: leading the way to quality care. *Nursing Times Learning Curve* **2**(4): 14–15.

Winstanley, F. (1996) Evaluation on site. *Primary Health Care* **6**(1): 11–12.

Appendix 1:
The Nurse Prescribers'
Formulary

The *Nurse Prescribers' Formulary* (NPF) forms an appendix to the *British National Formulary* (BNF). The products that nurses may prescribe are taken from 12 chapters of the BNF. The types of preparations that are included in the NPF are:

- laxatives
- analgesics
- local anaesthetics
- drugs for the mouth
- drugs for the removal of earwax
- drugs for threadworms
- drugs for scabies and head lice
- skin preparations
- agents for disinfection and cleansing
- wound management products
- elastic hosiery
- urinary catheters and appliances
- stoma care products
- appliances and reagents for diabetes
- fertility and gynaecological products.

Appendix 2:
Circumstances in which a nurse may prescribe

The NHS Executive HQ *Nurse Prescribing Guidance* April 1997 very clearly states, in Section 7, the circumstances in which nurses may prescribe. These are as follows:

Issues common to all nurse prescribers

7.1 Nurses qualified to prescribe cannot issue prescriptions on behalf of a practice nurse who is not a prescriber.

Prescriptions generated by a non-prescribing nurse must be presented to a GP to sign

7.2 Nurses can only write prescriptions on a prescription pad bearing their own unique identifier number.

7.3 A nurse prescription should generally provide treatment for no more than one calendar month. However, nurses will need to ensure that the prescription is cost effective and meets the clinical needs of the patient.

> *Patients requiring long term treatments will have their needs continually assessed and prescriptions issued should reflect assessed need. Only sufficient supplies should be prescribed to enable the fulfilment of the care plan, normally up to the re-evaluation date.*

7.4 Nurse prescriptions *must not* be written when an item has been administered to a patient using surgery stock; the cost of these items is already covered through the indirect reimbursement of practice expenses/Trust contracts respectively.

7.5 Nurses are not entitled to prescribe items which are not listed in the Secretary of State's list for nurse prescribing. This is published as Part XVIIB of the Drug Tariff and as an Appendix to the British National Formulary. Nurses may only prescribe in the manner in which they are set out in the prescribable list.

7.6 When a nurse becomes aware that the patient intends having a prescription dispensed by approaching an appliance contractor the nurse must ensure that the prescription does not contain medicinal preparations. *Appliance contractors cannot dispense medicinal preparations.*

7.7 Nurse prescribers may only issue prescriptions for the patients of the GP practices *covered by the health authority or GP contracts with the Trust. Nurses should not prescribe for others such as visiting relatives unless temporary registration with such a doctor has been arranged.*

7.8 Nurse prescribers must ensure that patients and clients are fully informed of the change in nursing responsibilities. Items available on nurse and GP prescription should be fully explained to ensure that there is no delay in obtaining supplies.

7.9 *Practice Nurse with District Nurse or Health Visitor Qualifications*

The practice nurse may prescribe in the GP surgery or in the home for the patients of the practice. The nurse should be mindful of any practice prescribing protocols and should only initiate a course of prescriptions after appropriately assessing the patient's needs.

7.10 The Department strongly advises that no more than six repeat prescriptions should be made, or six months elapse, whichever is the less, without reassessing the patient's needs.

7.11 The nurse may issue a repeat prescription on behalf of another nurse, provided that the other nurse is also registered as a nurse prescriber but the nurse must be sure that this is acceptable clinical practice because the clinical responsibility rests with the prescriber.

7.12 Items for dispensing on the practice nurse lilac form must only be those from the Secretary of State's list for nurse prescribers.

7.13 Items that are not in the Nurse Prescriber's List should not be entered on form FP10PN even if they are countersigned by a GP.

7.14 *District Nurses and Health Visitors*

District nurses and health visitors may prescribe in the surgery, the community clinic or in the home.

A district nurse who is qualified to prescribe may sign prescriptions for members of the district nursing team for patients on the caseload whom the district nurse has seen and whose treatment the nurse has initially assessed.

A prescribing district nurse may also sign a prescription when providing 'cover' for another prescribing district nurse who has originally seen the patient and assessed the treatment needed. It is important to note however, that whoever signs the prescription assumes responsibility *and the clinical liability for it*. In all cases, nurses must put themselves in a position to assess the necessity for, and appropriate choice of, drug, dressing or appliance before prescribing.

The nurse should be mindful of any prescribing protocols agreed within the GP practice relevant to the patient.

7.15 When a district nurse or health visitor who is qualified to prescribe is providing 'cover' for an absent colleague, who is also qualified to prescribe, the nurse providing cover may prescribe in their own right following a patient assessment and they may write a repeat prescription. Most community units have standards for reassessment periods and these may need to be reviewed in the light of nurse prescribing.

7.16 When a community district nurse or health visitor who works in a health clinic as cover for a practice nurse on behalf of the GP, the prescriptions written by the community district nurse or health visitor cannot be charged to the practice budget. This is because the nurse is not directly employed by the GP. Arrangements must be made within the contract to ensure that the contract for these services covers such occasions and that the resources required to reflect these arrangements are built into the Trust's notional budget. This will ensure that the community nurse can prescribe and the expenditure is reflected against the Trust budget.

7.17 Items for dispensing on the DN/HV green form must only be those from the Secretary of State's list for nurse prescribers.

7.18 Items that require a GP signature should not be entered on this form even if they are countersigned by the GP. (NHS Executive HQ 1997, pp. 13–16)

It is the responsibility of all nurse prescribers to familiarise themselves with and to observe the above regulations regarding nurse prescribing at all times. This is in the interest of good patient/client care and of safe and effective clinical practice.

Index